"The journey of recovery is more like a marathon than a sprint. In the book *The Recovery Cycle*, Joi Andreoli offers an in-depth and practical understanding of how addicted individuals can sustain the stamina needed for a marathon and successfully negotiate the twists and turns of the journey to lead a 'satisfied life' filled with an overall sense of wellbeing. Joi is a wonderful coach who allows individuals ways to examine important dimensions of recovery: thinking, decisions, feelings, choices, and connections with self and others. Her chapters are filled with wisdom gained from her personal journey blended with insights and sage advice about how to create and sustain a meaningful life from Carl Jung, David Burns, Viktor Frankl and many others. SAMHSA has defined recovery as 'a process of change through which individuals improve their health and wellness, live a self-directed life, and strive to reach their full potential.' The explorations and exercises in each chapter encourage all of us and our clients to dive deeper into this process of change, challenge our myths and self-deceptions, and use the helpful strategies offered to manage all the pitfalls and potholes along the journey. What a gem of a book. One that could be used by all who are seeking to break the cycle of addiction and live this self-directed life."

Carlo C. DiClemente, PhD, ABPP, *Emeritus Professor of Psychology, University of Maryland Baltimore County, author of* Addiction and Change: How Addictions Develop and Addicted People Recover

"*The Recovery Cycle* provides a much-needed shift in attitude and approach for people struggling to get sober from *any* addiction. Andreoli skillfully breathes new life into age-old concepts that are still effective while simultaneously inviting the reader to imagine their preferred life. The author ushers in a new era of addiction treatment by constructing a positive approach to the 12-Step Program. A must read for both recovering people and therapists alike!"

Alexandra Katehakis, PhD, *author of* Mirror of Intimacy: Daily Reflections on Emotional and Erotic Intelligence

"Beautifully written, engaging, inspirational—a love song to the freedom, creativity, and ever-evolving joys of recovery."

Katherine Ketcham, *co-author of* The Spirituality of Imperfection, Under the Influence *and* Broken

"A great book for therapists, their clients and anyone who wants a practical approach for recovery from any addiction. *The Recovery Cycle* shows how a meaningful recovery with connection and love can be simple, straightforward and attainable."

Dr. Pat Allen, CAS, *Psychotherapist, author of* It's a Man's World and a Woman's Universe

"Full of practical guidance, *The Recovery Cycle* is sure to be an asset to anyone seeking a deeply fulfilling recovery from addiction."

Julie S. Kraft, LMFT, *co-author of* The Mindfulness Workbook for Addiction *and* The Gift of Recovery

The Recovery Cycle

This book introduces the Recovery Cycle, the only relatable model for positive change in sobriety and a simple roadmap for sober living. The author, a clinician in recovery herself, demonstrates how to talk to clients or anyone with an interest in sobriety in a pragmatic, like-minded way.

The easy, conversational style encourages cultivation of solid, sober relationships and spiritual connections, all with an achievable, open-minded approach. Concrete methods honor the thinking and feeling parts of the recovering individual, thereby promoting personal empowerment and choice rather than generic prescriptive advice. The book speaks to all addiction disorders and discusses what every addicted person must go through to love their sober life, no matter what program they choose, no matter what addiction. Readers will find the journey toward emotional sobriety and spiritual recovery discussed in a simple, straightforward way, with depth and compassion.

For clinicians who want to guide clients in recovery or for any motivated individual in recovery desiring to transform their life from one of pain and struggle to a beautiful work of heart, this book will be a welcome spark of inspiration and support—without the snore factor of a dry textbook.

Joi Andreoli, LMFT, is a licensed marriage and family therapist, writer, and communications educator in the Los Angeles area.

The Recovery Cycle

A Practical Guide to Loving
Your Sober Life

Joi Andreoli

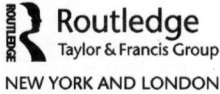
Routledge
Taylor & Francis Group

NEW YORK AND LONDON

First published 2023
by Routledge
605 Third Avenue, New York, NY 10158

and by Routledge
4 Park Square, Milton Park, Abingdon, Oxon, OX14 4RN

Routledge is an imprint of the Taylor & Francis Group, an informa business

Library of Congress Cataloging-in-Publication Data
Names: Andreoli, Joi (Therapist), author.
Title: The recovery cycle : a practical guide to loving your sober life /
   Joi Andreoli, LMFT.
Description: New York, NY : Routledge, 2023. | Includes bibliographical
   references and index.
Identifiers: LCCN 2022011849 (print) | LCCN 2022011850 (ebook) |
   ISBN 9781032275451 (hbk) | ISBN 9781032275444 (pbk) |
   ISBN 9781003293231 (ebk)
Subjects: LCSH: Addicts—Rehabilitation. | Addicts—Psychology. |
   Substance abuse—Treatment. | Compulsive behavior.
Classification: LCC RC564 .A526 2023 (print) | LCC RC564 (ebook) |
   DDC 362.29—dc23/eng/20220329
LC record available at https://lccn.loc.gov/2022011849
LC ebook record available at https://lccn.loc.gov/2022011850

ISBN: 978-1-032-27545-1 (hbk)
ISBN: 978-1-032-27544-4 (pbk)
ISBN: 978-1-003-29323-1 (ebk)

DOI: 10.4324/9781003293231

Typeset in Goudy
by Apex CoVantage, LLC

Contents

Preface

When I envisioned this book, my goal was to show precisely how readers could insert themselves into recovery and make the shift from an addictive hell to a sober, earthly heaven. In recovery, the heart, mind, and beyond all become areas of unlimited exploration and expansion. This change is a process that becomes a kind of transcendental journey. To some of you, this may sound like a lofty endeavor better suited to ancient yogis in the Himalayas, or perhaps more akin to a mind-blowing psychedelic trip, but without the hallucinogens.

Recovery is not a solitary practice of alienation and contemplation, though. Most of us aren't monks in the mountains. Nor is it an ever-present, colorful state of awesome connectedness (although glimpses of this may shimmer now and again). And recovery is neither dull nor a certain turn down "Gloom and Doom Street." Recovery, with all of its mystery, is a way to live with the knowable and unknowable, with mistakes and successes, with heart and mind—all without the drug or compulsive behavior. Recovering people know how to live life in a way that no matter what the feeling or circumstance, there can be a positive connection to others and to what is here right now; and yes, to what is beyond (and presumed for a select few gurus or acid excursions).

It seems any time is a time for spiritual healing and transformation back to individual and collective health. As societies evaluate their health and respond to public health crises, domestic divisions, and global challenges (and all the big issues that traverse time), recovering individuals, too, can take an inventory of their lives and make restorative adjustments for their own well-being. This focus on one's own recovery can transform the world. As Walter Russell said, "Each man is . . . empowered to uplift all men, as each drop of water uplifts the entire ocean."[1]

So how does anyone suffering from addiction heal and become a sober wave in this great ocean of life?

My answer to this question began in a graduate class. One of my professors was describing the Addiction Cycle on a whiteboard, and in my mind's eye, I saw another cycle coalesce—the Recovery Cycle—a positive mirror image of the Addiction Cycle.

I imagined the Recovery Cycle as a simple tool for transformation from addiction to wholeness—a compass of sorts.

Anyone can learn about a compass, but not everyone wants to use a compass to navigate through life, especially when it comes to relationships and emotions. Many rely on brain power alone to figure it out. This is especially true if there is an adventure with emotional risks on the horizon.

Many addicts have had their hearts severely broken. Opening one's heart and risking having it smashed even more can drive an addict's every thought and action into guarding his heart. Yet the recovering person's journey requires we take emotional risks. I believe we are better off taking such risks with a reliable compass. Relying on limited and often distorted thinking seems to be a continuous circle back to the murky waters of addiction or a dry sobriety.

The question of how to teach anyone to open their heart is something that seems to be in the realm of divine providence. To open one's heart is almost miraculous for the heart-guarded sort, especially for those who have experienced heartbreaking trauma.

We all have a story, and here is part of mine that I think is relevant to this heart stuff.

My brother, in the middle of the COVID-19 pandemic, was diagnosed with throat cancer and had a laryngectomy. Now, he has no vocal cords and breathes solely through a hole in his throat. Basically, he can't speak; he has no voice. Last year he finished treatment for prostate cancer, and in the last 10 years, he has had five hip surgeries.

The heart in me at the time of his throat surgery wanted to go visit him and rub his feet and joke with him, which, over the last 10 years, I have done because I wanted to. Logic at that time, though, right at the worst of the pandemic, voted on the side of safety. It was too risky. This decision was made knowing I (and the rest of my family) might not see him again. Many families have experienced similar realities.

My heart hurts over all of this. But I am glad it does.

Because of the pain in my chest, I know I feel deeply for this brother whom I didn't see for the better part of 25 years and with whom I was so angry for so long. Although sober now, he has been in and out of rehabs over many years for his own addictions, which for a very long time, I vehemently resented. *I got sober, why couldn't he?*

Among my many grudges, I believed he robbed the world of his astonishing musical talent. He's played guitar brilliantly by ear all of his life, alone in his room. I wanted to see him share this incredible gift. His playing seemed to be his way of communicating to our family, "Hear me, I exist."

When I was a teenager, I often wanted him to just go away. Amplified wailings would spill out of his room into mine, disrupting my silent study time. I hated him and his disregard. Later I would understand my brain couldn't appreciate what was going on with him. It was too busy fending off my own demons.

If I were still using, or sober and dry, I would be bitter. I know it. My heart wouldn't be feeling anything except hard. My brain would be telling you a very different story of resentment and victimhood; it would be blaming the childhood trauma, the parents, the way the waitress raised her eyebrow, the expired milk in the fridge, my brother, and his blaring guitar.

I see myself kind of like the Tin Man in *The Wizard of Oz* who wanted a heart. I didn't realize I actually had one all along. My heart was right there in my chest for years, well into my sobriety, saying, "I'm in here! Free me!" One day, it occurred to me my heart wasn't a lost junkyard scrap after all, but a living thing with an ever-increasing capacity for love. Today, my heart feels almost too big for my body.

The point? It is truly miraculous that old beliefs and grievances have vanished. I feel love for my brother, family, others, and the world I did not think possible. This miracle is available for any recovering person who is willing to take a risk on the odyssey known as recovery.

This book, then, will describe the Recovery Cycle (which can be understood through the brain) and will also show how recovering people take emotional risks, feel feelings, and love themselves and others better (the heart part).

In recovery, our hearts will feel a lot of things and will ultimately heal with a balanced blend of the pragmatic and spiritual. The brain and heart, with good guidance, can work and heal together. With this, we will move beyond petty gripes and profound challenges, families will heal, and societies will improve.

The whole of humanity's wellness depends upon all of us living and loving better in connected, healthy relating. For those of us in recovery, we have a tool to do just that—the Recovery Cycle.

Recovery During a Pandemic and Anytime

What could those suffering from addiction use during a pandemic, or anytime really?

- Methods for how to transcend confusion, fear, and disorientation.
- Time to stretch and think beyond habitual, distorted thought patterns.
- Information about how a lifetime of love and healthy relationships is possible and doable.
- A simple road map for connection and wholeness.

As we come out of the pandemic, addicts everywhere are still experiencing serious challenges. Tension at home, aching isolation, depression, relapse, communication problems, safety issues, and more add up to a lot of stress for both addicted and recovering people (not to mention those who might fall prey to addiction). I've heard a few people say their twisted and obsessive thinking has them contemplating suicide.

A swelling despair and loneliness addicts know so well—even without a pandemic—can whirl into overwhelming proportions, spinning like a black hole only to cave in on itself, swallowing up the addict's very existence (meanwhile consuming other vulnerable ones into a dark space of their own). The addict brain, roaming alone, is not a fun zone. Especially now.

As a recovering person myself, I admit my brain can go to gloomy places too, that is, when I leave it alone for too long. There is one synaptic bright spot, however, which I seek out on a daily basis and wholeheartedly embrace.

Recovery from addiction is attainable and can be joyful and meaningful, no matter what the circumstance or what contagion is on deck. This is the Recovery Cycle's promise and what this book is about.

Work Cited

Clark, Glenn. *The Man Who Tapped the Secrets of the Universe*. 20th ed. Waynesboro, VA: University of Science and Philosophy, 2008.

Acknowledgments

First, I want to acknowledge and express my deep gratitude to Dr. Pat Allen. Years spent in conversation with Dr. Allen gave me tremendous insight into how people can live a balanced, love-filled life—if we do the personal work. Dr. Allen's infinite supply of support has assisted me in honoring my own Recovery Cycle and sharing it with you.

Also, Dr. Allen's signature WANT® training program instructs people on how to communicate with personal integrity and authenticity to achieve their life goals. Learning this system with all of the WANT® training students is one of the highlights of my journey, and I am grateful for all of the scholastic ideas and intimate details shared in class with fellow students.

I extend my deep gratitude to Ann Hale Bailey, for her enduring friendship since day one of my sobriety and for modeling how to live a spiritual life in recovery; Geoffry D. White, PhD, for his encouragement of raw first drafts and endnote conversations; Denise Dexter Buckner, for her spot-on comments and so much more; Mario DeSalvo, LMFT, professor extraordinaire, who helped shaped more than he knows; Andrea Frazer, for her humor, editing experience, and urging me on. I also want to thank Tammy Nelson, PhD, Douglas Moser, and Jeff Hume-Pratuch, for their professional support and encouragement, as well as Alexandra Katehakis, PhD and Jerry Saslow, LMFT, for their valuable insights and input.

And, of course, I want to acknowledge all the individuals and couples in recovery I've had the pleasure of meeting over the years. Thank you for sharing your pain and joys with me.

Finally, to my husband and family for providing the space for me to grow in love and intimacy; I am beyond grateful for the recovery and love we all share.

Note

1. Glenn Clark, *The Man Who Tapped the Secrets of the Universe*, 20th ed. (Waynesboro, VA: University of Science and Philosophy, 2008), 48.

Introduction

Reading this book, you will be transported into the world of addiction and recovery. From the beginning, I want you, the clinician, to step into your client's shoes and walk the recovery walk. From the start, I will also ask you, whether you be a counselor, mental health professional, or clergy (all of whom many clients consider "Oz," in a sense), to identify in a way where you can feel true empathy for the sufferer who struggles to stay clean and sober. How to do this?

To truly empathize, I will ask you to think of a substance or behavior that has been a problem for you in some way—a compulsive activity that messes with your well-being or equanimity. Choose something—it can be anything, maybe something from your past if nothing is a problem for you now—where you've been obsessed with getting more, where a little too much of your mental attention is spent preoccupied with obtaining that person, love, thing, or activity you've got to have. Maybe it's salty popcorn every night, or excessive purchases of clothing, or . . .? Ultimately, the idea is, you suspect the object (or activity) of your desire isn't good for you, or may not be. A little voice inside you knows it.

Then, the bulk of each chapter will mostly be me, as a therapist and recovering person, talking directly to you, the reader, who has the addiction affliction. In this way, this book is written for you and those who want relief from addiction (or a lackluster sobriety).

As you read along, maybe with your client, if you've suggested this book as bibliotherapy (which I highly recommend), you may experience that wonderful combo of empathy, compassion, and lightheartedness—the mixed flavor of emotion that seems to act as the spoonful of sugar to help the medicine of the work in recovery go down.

Also, whatever your client's (or your) affliction, you can settle into the Clinician's Corner at each chapter's end. This area offers exercises to aid in your client's healing and will be useful to you as well with your (past or present) affliction. Here, I suggest you do the exercises to gain more of that empathy, compassion, and lightheartedness about the process of becoming a sober, self-actualized human being, which is what recovery is all about.

DOI: 10.4324/9781003293231-1

So now, identify the thing you want to abstain from as you read this book. Consider this thing your addiction. Now, think of the worst consequence you experienced with your addiction. After you've felt the feelings (which I bet don't feel good), proceed.

Are You Ready to Kiss Your Addiction Goodbye?

If you've picked up this book, you've most likely encountered a rough road with your addiction. There's a good chance you're at the point in life where if drinking, using, or engaging in that behavior was fun, free, and easy all of the time, you'd still be doing it. But you're not. You're here, right now, reading this Introduction. And as unbelievable as it might sound right now, living a fun, free life without your drug or that compulsive behavior is possible and doable.

If Recovery Seems Impossible for You, Read On

Whatever your addiction and whatever difficulty you've experienced, my hope for you is that you will come to know that recovery can be made simple and is easily available. Think about your last fling with your drug (or compulsive activity) for a moment. How was it coming down after your fix? From what I know, staying drug free will always be easier than the comedown or undeniable consequences of the last bender (and probably easier than managing, controlling, and keeping secrets around your addiction as well).

A Simple Plan for a Complicated You

Like most addicts, you're likely complicated. It's normal to feel overwhelmed at the notion of a clean, sober life. Relax if you can. You will find in this book a simple plan for recovery. You will find in these pages a straightforward, easy process for getting and staying sober. This book will walk you through the process, and you will come to know the Recovery Cycle as your friendly guide. If you choose recovery, your friendly guide (this book) and other good friends will meet you along the way.

A Little About Me

I am a recovering person who has been over 40 years sober from alcohol and all mind-altering chemicals. I qualify for a few other addictions as well, including codependence, but thanks to living the Recovery Cycle, I'm leading a fun, free, exciting life without substances and compulsive people pleasing. I am also a marriage and family therapist. In my work and personal life, I see firsthand the power of healthy relationships in recovery. With a continued Recovery Focus, I live a satisfied, creative, love-filled life rooted in relationships. When people feel connected, they transform. You can too.

Why I Wrote This Book

I wrote this book to show addicted people precisely how they can insert themselves into their own recovery program and what to expect living as a clean and sober person. Becoming familiar with what recovery entails is the beginning of an easier life that can be filled with relief, love, meaning, and even awe. This is what the Recovery Cycle is all about.

Why Read This Book?

One reason to read this book is to discover how you can heal from addiction and create a solid recovery that works for you. Also, you will see what you can expect living a drug-free life. Most important, the Recovery Cycle supports how YOU choose to experience your sober journey and live the life you want.

Does This Sound Too Good to Be True?

The recovery process as outlined in this book is a simple and easy plan, but some days being sober may not feel easy. That's okay. This book will help you navigate your feelings as you create your own personal plan in spite of any difficulties you might experience. And isn't that really the only way to truly learn something? To do it yourself with supportive guidance?

Live a Joyful Life

You can live a joyful life. Living substance free or not engaging in compulsive activity is not about giving up pleasure, fun, laughter, and creativity. In fact, the opposite is true. I've found the door flies open every time I've made a real attempt to discover the joys and good feelings of life. Together, let's make your recovery simple so you can live easier. Your easy, custom-made recovery plan awaits. Want to start designing now?

How to Use This Book

This book is written for clinicians and the person recovering from addiction. Therefore, for reasons already stated, I will mainly be talking to the recoverer (á la one addict talking to another). That said, you might be a clinician, student, client, or anyone else with an interest in recovery. For now, however, on this journey, think of being a person in recovery.

As you may know, recovery doesn't happen overnight or with a quick read of any book. Recovery must be lived over time. We gather information over time and then apply what we learn. We aren't computers and cannot simply download recovery into our brains. We are human. Recovery takes time.

Take Your Time

Take as long as you like to read each chapter and see what fits and where you identify. You may want to keep a special notebook or journal if anything comes up for you. Take the time to discover who you are in recovery.

Pronouns Explained

On occasion I use the pronoun *he*. The use of *he* is in no way representative of, or adhering to, any patriarchal ideology. This book is for all who want to heal from addiction or any compulsive behavior, whether identifying as she/he/they/them or any neopronoun.

Addiction—and recovery—do not discriminate.

The pronoun *we* is used on occasion. As I am a recovering person, I include myself with you on this journey.

Other Nomenclature Notes

Addict: The term "addict" is used on occasion, which is not meant to stigmatize. Many sufferers self-identify as addicts, as I do, so I use it for simplicity and an easier read. If you don't like the term, please replace it with any word that works for you.

Using: At times, I use the term "using" for substance abuse and compulsive behavior. This means, for example, if I say a gambler "uses," I mean the using is gambling.

Sex addiction: As clinicians may know, sex addiction is not listed in the *DSM-5*. Also, some mental health professionals see sexual compulsivity as simply a maladaptive response—not in the category of addiction. My thought? One can consider repeated sexual behavior that causes harm an addiction, a maladaptive response, compulsive sexual behavior, acting out sexually, or whatever you want to call it. This book, in short, takes a neutral stance on what you want to call continued compulsive sexual behavior that harms one's life.

The Recovery Cycle, with all of the different opinions and words out there, is mainly concerned with what to do instead of engaging in addictive substances or addictive-like behaviors—including sexual compulsivity—that hurt, cause harm, and are rife with negative consequences.

For Skimmers

At the end of each chapter you will see a "Recovery Recap." This recap highlights the key points of each chapter.

Also, you will see some sentences bolded throughout each chapter—these are important callouts, so while skimming you can easily see these main points.

Clinician's Corner

At the end of each chapter, you will find exercises in the Clinician's Corner section. The exercises are for clinicians to give clients or for question prompts in individual or group sessions. The exercises stimulate healing and serve to raise consciousness about one's own part in addiction and recovery. Written responses are suggested. Writing can be like taking medicine to get well from a serious illness. Healing may be accelerated by answering the questions in writing.[1]

"Straight Shot" shorter exercises live in the clinician's area. If you sense the long version may be too much at any time, use the Straight Shot.

Important notes for clinicians: It is not a good idea to press anyone to share what they don't want to share. This can be triggering, especially for those who have experienced trauma. Provide a safe space and see what happens. Also, I suggest you do the exercises before giving them to your client. This will help you with empathy.

QR Code and Video

At the end of each chapter, you will find a video of me, talking to you, for a quick minute. I offer some personal experience and a few nuggets of additional information in this wrap up.

A QR Code is how you will access the video, and it looks like this:

To access the video:

1. Simply open the camera app on your mobile phone, iPad, or smart device as if you were to take a picture.
2. Point your device at the code, centering the code on the screen until you see a web address pop up.
3. Click on the web address that you see on the screen.
4. Press play.

The QR code on this page includes links to all of the videos for this book. I look forward to seeing you there.

Additional Exercises

A few additional exercises are embedded in Chapters 3, 7, and 8 in boxes with a pencil icon. These will be especially helpful in galvanizing healing and growth.

Read in Order, or Not

Each chapter builds on the chapter before, so best to read the chapters in order. That said, the concepts could stand alone. Reading in a sequential way, however, will be more digestible; you will get more out of it, too, especially for those newer to recovery. (Or, for those who like to read the end first, go to Chapter 12 now and see what is in store for you.)

Read a Little—Read a Lot: It's Up to You

Keep in mind this book is an easy read—you can read little bits at a time or bigger chunks, whatever suits you. There is no rush in completing this book or how you choose to experience the Recovery Cycle. How you do your recovery is your choice.

Boxes You Won't Want to Miss

Boxes with text inside expand on an idea mentioned previously in the main text. All have good information about an important part of recovery.

Vignettes and Real-Life Experience, Anyone?

Vignettes are scattered throughout in grey boxes. To protect the privacy of the individuals, names have been changed, and circumstances from each vignette have been created from a blend of more than one person's real-life experience.

I share a bit about myself a few times as well. What I say about me is all true.

Secular, or Not

This Recovery Cycle does not require anyone to believe anything about religion, spirituality, or the secular. Individuals choose for themselves what works for them.

Endnotes

Created to lead motivated readers to stellar resources/bibliotherapy.

Support and Good Guides Help

Mental health professionals, counselors, and clients/people in recovery all need guidance at times, especially when it comes to addiction and recovery.

To the Mental Health Professional/Counselor

You as a clinician may be the first guide for your client. Although this book asks you to go on the journey with your client, you are the guide—it is all about them. Therefore (as you must already know), self-disclosure can come in small doses, if at all (depending on your theoretical orientation), and only if clinically relevant. If you have any confusion about this, seek supervision.

To People in Recovery

If you don't have a recovery guide (that one trustworthy person who supports you in your recovery), I strongly suggest you find one. This person is someone with whom you feel safe enough to be completely honest to share your findings. We can't do recovery alone.

Also, sharing your discoveries with other sober peers in a recovery program will help support you as well. One idea is to read this book with another sober friend (or with a group) and discuss how what you have read applies to your life in recovery.

If you choose a Twelve Step or other recovery program, regular attendance at meetings/gatherings will be vital. Many ideas in this book will come alive as you listen to others share their problems and solutions. The Recovery Cycle fits any good program.

Whoever you choose as your recovery support squad, remember: **No one can decide who you are and what is in your own heart.** No one person knows what is best for you in all things.

Note

1. James W. Pennebaker, *Writing to Heal: A Guided Journal for Recovering From Trauma and Emotional Upheaval* (Oakland, CA: New Harbinger Press, 2004), 3–16. Research indicates that writing about emotional upheaval and trauma can improve physical and mental health. This short book offers simple writing exercises and scientifically sound information about the specific benefits of expressive writing. As prescribed in Pennebaker's book, it is not necessary to share one's writing with anyone. Pennebaker suggests that positive results occur when one has the freedom to safely express oneself without a witness. Writing is an indispensable tool for healing in recovery, and Pennebaker's method is a wonderful resource for anyone who has experienced trauma, emotional upheaval, or shame around any secret. Consider it another tool for the recovery tool kit.

Work Cited

Pennebaker, James W. *Writing to Heal: A Guided Journal for Recovering From Trauma and Emotional Upheaval.* Oakland, CA: New Harbinger Press, 2004.

Part One

A Merry-Go-Round Prison

1   The Addiction Cycle

In This Chapter

* Am I Suffering From Addiction?
* Solitary Confinement
* Triggers and Cravings
* Reasons Addicts Are Different

I am a person, like you. And I happen to be a therapist who is sober—with a recovery solution.

If you are reading this, you must want some insight into recovery from addiction. You are most likely a therapist, or possibly a client of a therapist. Or, perhaps you are a person suffering from addiction—not ready to quit—but you like the idea of transformation. Or, maybe you are wondering how you can stop something or just cut back on that something. That something could be alcohol, drugs, sex, porn, gambling, sugar, or any other thing that might be causing a problem for you. And there are many things that can cause problems.

I have struggled with addiction to more than a few things. As a therapist and sober person, I've witnessed clients and others grapple with addiction. I've also watched and experienced the attendant fear and low self-esteem that seems to fuel addiction's fire. Over the years, though, I've also come to know recovery—intimately. But more on that as we go. So back to you.

I wrote this book to give you—mental health professionals—or anyone suffering from addiction—a simple way to look at how you can play a part in recovery. It is possible to move from a *seemingly* hopeless state of mind and body to meaningful purpose. Yes. This can be manifested with heaps of love, to boot. If you've experienced recovery, you know this is possible, especially with a "one addict talking to another" kind of dialogue. Sober speak inspires positive action and the space to freely breathe—it is the oxygen to recovery's clean air.

In the following pages, you will get to take in that air as you walk in the addict's shoes and discover the recovery walk.

In this guide, you will hear me talking directly to a person who may be suffering from addiction or stumbling in sobriety. You will also encounter some tricks of the therapist's trade. So, mental health people, get ready to slip on

DOI: 10.4324/9781003293231-3

your client's work boots as you gather more tools for your therapist's tool belt. And addiction sufferers? Well, remember in *The Wizard of Oz* when Dorothy pulled back that curtain and found . . . a person? That person is me, and that person is you, too. Nothing to be afraid of. No tricks here. Only touchstones and questions laid out in the open for you to make your sober life what you want it to be.

Finding home—*your original state of wholeness*—may take more than clicking your heels together, but that's okay. You will find your own way, just as Dorothy did. She went back to Kansas, her home. But not everyone wants to live in Kansas, on that farm, in that house. You get to be you, which is what a good therapist will help you do.

Now, let's get started.

Am I Suffering From Addiction?

If you don't know the answer to this question, keep reading this chapter and see if anything rings true for you. There are definitions and questionnaires specific to any addiction you can find online, too. Typically, though, **people who are not addicts don't think about whether or not they have a problem**. Some people, too, are in denial about their addiction and stay oblivious in spite of all the negative consequences. Those people probably aren't reading this book.

But before even saying you are addicted to something, or admitting you are an addict, let's take a brief look at what addiction looks like.

Note: As we proceed, keep in mind the term *addict* will be used on occasion throughout this book to describe anyone addicted to anything (i.e., substance related or a compulsive behavior) and whether still using/engaging in the addictive activity, abstinent only, or abstinent and in recovery. The term is not meant to stigmatize; it is used as some addicts in recovery commonly use it. If you don't like its usage, feel free to replace it with any other term that works for you.

Solitary Confinement

The addict lives in a self-constructed prison. The prison, though, is like some absurd carnival theme park, where the addict chains himself to the addiction merry-go-round and experiences a kind of perpetual solitary confinement—a seemingly never-ending state of isolation where he spins behind walls of illusion and fantasy. At times he feels dizzyingly high, while other times, not so much. The not-so-much part is a kind of bizarre, ghastly hell. If you are an addict, you know this strange, dark, limiting netherworld all too well. Pain seems to dog you at every corner, except for those moments of relief when the high kicks in.

There was a time when I had an addiction to Entenmann's chocolate chip cookies. This may sound funny, and granted, this wasn't as serious as the alcohol and cocaine addiction I knew in my teen years, but it was painful, nonetheless.

My dirty little secret. A way to avoid my own pain, anxiety, and despair. This was *after* I sobered up from alcohol and drugs.

I fantasized about the bite-sized goodies during the day, resisting their charms, until nighttime when I would give in and head out to the grocery store to purchase the little buggers. If you are an addict, you might guess that most of the cookies were devoured by the time I returned home. Then, I would finish the box off that night, vowing *never again*, only to start dreaming about them by noon the next day.

With the cookies (as with the alcohol and cocaine) my very soul felt irretrievable. I didn't know who or what was taking over my body and mind. I wasn't me, but I was me. I often felt like a shell of a person. A person impersonating a person. Over and over again.

This isolating, round-and-round experience can apply to any addiction, whether the addiction is alcohol, sex, gambling, Entenmann's devil cookies, or anything else. It is an actual cycle—the Addiction Cycle.

The Addiction Cycle has four parts, but before we get to our textbook definition, let's look more closely at how these four parts play out for, let's say, an ice cream addict. If you are wondering if you have an addiction problem, just replace the ice cream with your drug (or behavior) of choice. Granted, ice cream is not the same as meth or heroin; this example is not meant to discount any addiction but to illustrate in a lighter way what you may already know is deeply painful. (If you are an overeater that's ever had a sugar hangover, however, the ice cream addiction won't seem funny at all.)

The Ice Cream Addict

Preoccupation: This person loves peppermint ice cream and thinks about eating it a lot. Throughout the day and often, he thinks about the moment he can lie on the couch and eat his big, dreamy bowl of pink ice cream. He thinks about where he will purchase his ice cream, what favorite bowl he will use to eat his favorite ice cream, when he will eat the ice cream (after dinner), and what show he will watch as he eats the ice cream.

Rituals: This person now leaves work and goes to the store he knows has his special brand of peppermint ice cream. With feigned nonchalance he wanders in the store and goes to the produce section first. As usual, he decides to purchase something other than ice cream so no one will know he is there just for the ice cream. Once home, he eats a big dinner and makes sure, as customary, that he eats the produce he bought so he gets nutrients in his body before eating the ice cream. He tidies up the kitchen before getting his favorite bowl out of the cupboard, as he usually does. As he does all these things, he feels the charge of getting high, knowing his ice cream is just a few feet away in the freezer.

Using: Now, on the couch, he is binging on the peppermint ice cream. He is totally blissed out and strangely relieved while eating the ice cream. Everything is okay in that moment. He finishes the gallon.

Despair: The next morning, he wakes up with a massive sugar hangover, feeling guilty and shameful that he devoured the entire bucket. He planned to have only two scoops. Feeling demoralized and awfully alone with his secret he thinks, *I'm not going to eat ice cream ever again*. But, when the afternoon or the next week rolls around, he starts dreaming about peppermint ice cream one more time.

When you plug in your favorite substance or behavior, do you identify in any way?

Now let's take a look at that textbook definition. Remember from the "How to Use this Book" section that the word *using* throughout this text is the general stand-in word for using substances or engaging in compulsive behavior.

The Addiction Cycle

In Figure 1.1 you will see the four stages in the Addiction Cycle:[1]

1. *Preoccupation*: When the addict's thinking is completely obsessed with the substance, activity, or behavior. All thinking is geared toward the fantasy of what using will feel like. This fantasy propels the addict to the next stage.
2. *Rituals*: The routines or set of behaviors that lead up to Using. Rituals intensify the Preoccupation. The Rituals (behaviors) and Preoccupation (mindset) develop into somewhat of a feedback loop, until Using occurs. Once Rituals are engaged, it is almost inevitable that the addict will use. The chemical reaction in the body is jump-started here—the addict often feels high during this phase.
3. *Using*: The ingestion of the substance (e.g., the alcoholic takes a drink) or engagement in behavior (e.g., the sex addict engages in another hookup). A chemical reaction in the body is in full swing here.
4. *Despair*: The despair, shame, and guilt felt after Using. These feelings are the result of using, but more specifically come from: breaking one's vow to never use again; the physiological comedown from the substance/behavior; and the absolute powerlessness the addict experiences around the Using.

For relief from the increasingly intense negative feelings of shame and guilt, the addict eventually becomes preoccupied once again, focusing on the fantasy of good feelings the next round of using promises to fulfill. Thus, he manages his way back to Preoccupation in the cycle.

In other instances, he vows to never use again and temporarily forgets the profound shame of his last binge. He rationalizes that there isn't a problem and so becomes preoccupied with the fantasy of using one more time.

Isolation: You'll see underneath Using is Isolation. In brief, anytime addicts use, they put themselves further and further away from a true connection to themselves and others. Addicts know this to their core. They are starkly isolated and often feel freakishly alone with shame.

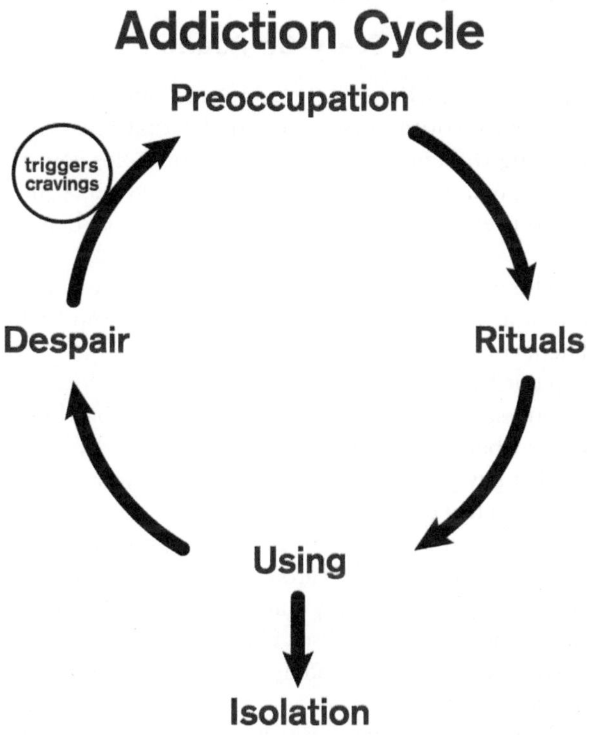

Addiction Cycle

Preoccupation

triggers cravings

Despair

Rituals

Using

Isolation

Figure 1.1 The Addiction Cycle.

A Merry-Go-Round That Isn't Merry

If you've ever experienced this cycle, you know the feeling of being out of control, demoralized, lonely, and most likely a little (or a lot) frightened. Whatever your addiction, even if peppermint ice cream, you may think that what started out as fun and harmless somehow morphed into a ghoulish prison park nightmare.

You may remember climbing on the merry-go-round carousel with the other kids with a child-like innocence and sense of wonder and excitement, but now, older, you are stuck amidst scary mannequin horses, still grasping for that brass ring. The park closed a long time ago, but there you are, stuck going round and round, all alone and in the dark, except for the other soulless, glass-eyed creatures going around with you. You may wonder why you can't just forget about that brass ring and step off the merry-go-round and go home. But you just can't, because there it is, coming around again, that brass ring full of promise, begging you to try and grab it one more time.

At this point, you may totally get what the Addiction Cycle is all about. Maybe you've lived it. If so, skip ahead to "Triggers and Cravings." If you want more though, see "A Scary-Go-Round."

A Scary-Go-Round

Preoccupation: This is where you imagine your carousel fantasy. You see yourself on your favorite horse, reaching for that brass ring, grabbing it, and winning the big prize. This fantasy occupies your thinking to an intense degree, and you play it over and over in your head. You can't help yourself and feel compelled to make your brass ring dream come true.

Rituals: This is when you ritually go online to see where there is a merry-go-round. You find one, because you always can find one somewhere. Then, you make your preparations:

You map out how to get to the theme park. You dress in your usual loose clothing so you can comfortably reach for that brass ring. You know exactly what you will do when you get there—how you will joke with the ticket guy and what you will look for in your horse. As you do these things, you feel dizzyingly high.

Using: You step on to the merry-go-round and find the special white horse you imagined earlier. The carousel starts going around and around; you feel so giddy you can hardly stand it. Then, you see the object of your dreams—the brass ring. Closer. Closer. Then, you reach for the ring . . . but miss it. You try again and again. But again and again, your big fingers miss it.

Despair: Now you feel down—no, despair—realizing for the trillionth time that the brass ring will never be yours. It is made for children's fingers, not your adult-size paw. The carousel slows, and the guilt and shame you feel are unbearable as you slump and hide behind your white horse. The awful feelings are compounded even more when you see the carousel operator closing up for the night, leaving you all alone with your favorite fiberglass horse and the other marble-eyed animals stuck on the merry-go-round with you. In spite of the carousel company, you feel pathetically alone.

But strangely, after the sun comes up and the afternoon rolls around, you start fantasizing all over again. You think that another carousel, or, maybe a stationary horse, would get you closer to that brass ring.

Triggers and Cravings

If you look at Figure 1.1 again, you will also see "Triggers" and "Cravings" to the top left. If you are unfamiliar with these terms, here's what these words mean:

Triggers are anything that pulls an addict toward using. Triggers can be people, places, things, or feelings—anything that gets the addict hankering for the hit. Depending on the addiction, a trigger could be walking by the liquor or bread aisle, fighting with your spouse or child, feeling lonely, feeling happy, seeing a massage parlor on the boulevard, going to a wedding, seeing carousel horses or peppermint ice cream, and so on. As you might guess, triggers are personal and can be almost anything.

Cravings are well, *CRAVINGS*. This is when the body feels an extreme need for the drug or behavior coupled with persistent thoughts like, "I *NEED* it *NOW*" or "Gotta have it."[2] If you have ever craved, you get the point. It's like having an outbreak of poison oak or chicken pox with that itch that *NEEDS* scratching. You might go crazy if you couldn't scratch that itch.

Beware of triggers and cravings because:

Triggers and cravings, when not consciously dealt with, can hook the addict into the Addiction Cycle.

Have you ever been triggered and then become mentally obsessed with getting your fix? Have you ever had cravings? Has this obsession felt like an uncontrollable urge in your body that you couldn't will away?

More on Cravings

An addict will do practically anything to get their drug of choice and then do crazy things to get more. There never seems to be enough. Can you think of something you've done to get your drug that is completely uncharacteristic of who you think you are? And once engaged in your addiction, could you stop midstream?

One thing we know for sure is that addiction is not about being weak willed. As addicts, we know we'll do whatever it takes to get our drug when we may want it—the cravings are just that intense. You might be wondering, as a lot of people addicted to something do, what is the reason for the overpowering compulsion to use that something? And how come other people don't have a problem with the craving part like we do? Why aren't we addicts like other people when it comes to that something we need NOW?

Reasons Addicts Are Different

One older idea about why addicts might be different from other people when it comes to addiction is the concept of an allergy.[3] As addicts know, it almost feels like an allergic reaction ignites when we are triggered into obsessively thinking about our chosen drug or behavior. The Preoccupation gets the body revved up, in a sense. Our bodies feel the craving. Then, with the rituals of using, the mind convinces the body to use. We intimately know this allergy-like condition because of how our insides feel, how we crave, and the uncontrollable nature of our experience when we want to scratch that craving itch.

The solution to avoiding an allergic reaction is to avoid the thing we are allergic to. If you are allergic to strawberries, you don't eat strawberries. You wouldn't go to Strawberries Anonymous or to rehab because you couldn't stop eating strawberries. You would just quit eating strawberries. But with our drug of choice, it seems almost impossible to just quit.

Although the intense craving sensation and compulsion may not be a pure medical example of an allergy, we can agree that something peculiar and abnormal transpires in the mind and body of a person when that mind and body are preoccupied with using. Many consider this peculiarity a disease, which more recent evidence supports.[4] (As a side note, Bill Wilson, cofounder of Alcoholics Anonymous, was wary of using the word disease and considered the disease concept an outside issue. He preferred the terms "illness" or "malady.")[5] Today, the American Medical Association, American Psychiatric Organization, the National Council on Alcoholism and Drug Dependence, and the World Health Organization consider alcoholism a disease.

Another more recent proposition is that addicts have a physiological/neurological susceptibility to addiction (and to their drug or behavior of choice). This theory, simply put, says the terrain of the "craving brain" is molded by a combo of genetics, hormones, and stress. The brain, through a complicated chain of events, can become vulnerable to addiction.[6]

Addiction Is More Than the Physiological

There is a lot more to what energizes addiction besides the science and physiological. Other players help give rise to the Addiction Cycle's shadowy hell show. Faulty belief systems, low self-esteem, fear stemming from childhood wounds, trauma, or other environmental factors often play starring roles in the drama as well. In general, though? Pain is a common denominator—with the pursuit of pleasure giving rise to compulsive consumption.[7] Typically, it is how those vulnerable to addiction deal with these issues (the pain), along with the physiological, that sets addicted people apart from those not addicted. We'll touch a little more on these ideas later.

Whatever the roots of addiction, addicts would probably all agree on one simple fact: We like how we feel when high. For many of us, using felt like it put us in a state of "normal."

This idea of feeling "normal" while using is especially true for opioid users.

> Prolonged and increasingly higher doses of opioids change the brain so that it functions more or less normally when the drug is present and abnormally when the drug is removed. That's why it's said a person with opioid addiction uses the drug in order to feel "normal."[8]

As said before, though, I think all addicts could identify with that "ahh, it's all good now" feeling of normal when it comes to their drug of choice. At some point, however, during what feels normal (until it doesn't), some people cross an invisible line into addiction, whether it be with a substance or behavior.

Another last thought here about what sets addicted people apart: There never seems to be enough of that something that gets us high.

All of the ideas and information out there about what makes addicts different and what fuels addiction's ferocious flames—the physical, emotional, psychological, and spiritual—are very good topics to explore. But if you have a problem with a substance or compulsive behavior and want to be free from your addiction, keep it simple. Quit one day or one minute at a time, reach out for help, and hang out with other people who have quit. Consider this analogy I heard a long time ago from an anonymous source:

If your pants are on fire, it is best not to sit there and ponder why your pants are on fire. Better to jump in the lake that is right next to you and put the fire out. Then, once the fire is out, you can figure out how your pants got on fire.

If your mind and body are burning from your drug, there is no chance for recovery until you quit and put the flame out. **Abstinence is a must for healing from addiction** and reclaiming a healthy body and sound mind.

Still Wondering If You Are an Addict?

If you're still haggling within yourself about quitting your thing, you might not be ready to take the action step (of abstinence) into recovery. Maybe you like the status quo, or possibly you are considering the value and need for change but feel ambivalent; or, maybe reading this book is you beginning to develop your action plan as you prepare for your new life.[9]

Ultimately, whether or not you are suffering from addiction—enough to abstain—is for you to decide and accept, but remember:

> **Recovery can only happen when you abstain from your drug of choice (or compulsive behavior).**

Are you ready to start your recovery now?

Recovery Recap

- The Addiction Cycle is the addict's prison and has four parts: Preoccupation, Rituals, Using, Despair.
- Isolation and an aching aloneness are guaranteed when you use.
- Triggers are anything that pulls the addict toward using. Triggers are people, places, things, and feelings.
- Cravings are when the body feels the extreme need for the drug or behavior, coupled with persistent thoughts like, "I need it NOW!"
- There are many ideas about what fuels addiction, all of which can be explored only if you are abstinent.

- Beware of triggers and cravings—when not consciously dealt with they can hook you back into the Addiction Cycle.
- Abstinence is a must for recovery and healing from addiction.
- Only you can decide if you are an addict and want recovery.
- Recovery is only possible when you abstain from your drug or compulsive behavior.

Clinician's Corner

If your client wonders if addiction might be a problem, describe the Addiction Cycle to them or have them read this chapter. Use a whiteboard or paper, if they don't have a copy of this book. (I use the equivalent of a giant Post-It plastered on the wall in my office.) Some people are visual learners, and the visual reinforces the learning. Ask the following questions (in the Addiction Cycle Inventory), either in your session or group, or copy the questions and give them to your client for homework. These instructions apply for each chapter going forward. The instructions are for you to give your client homework or in session work.

Also, if you—as a therapist and person—have ever had a problem with feeling addicted to anything, or if using a substance or engaging in any compulsive behavior was ever a problem for you, answer the questions. Maybe your addiction/compulsive behavior is a dating app, or other social media/technology overconsumption, or frozen yogurt. (Gabor Maté, author of *In the Realm of Hungry Ghosts: Close Encounters With Addiction,* had an addiction to classical CDs, so it can be anything.)[10] The best would be for you to give up that something (at least for two months) while you read this book. This will help you understand what it's like to be in your client's work boots.

Addiction Cycle Inventory (20–40 Minutes)

Review the Addiction Cycle (Figure 1.1) and write out your answers.

1. Triggers/cravings: List any triggers you might have and describe your cravings, if you have any. Remember: Triggers can be internal (feelings/thoughts) or external (things outside you). Triggers are personal. Cravings are an intense, uber-urgent, abnormal desire or longing for something. Not everyone has cravings.

2. Preoccupation: Write down how you used to think about using. This stage is about the fantasy. Your fantasies are personal. Write them all down. Also, do you still fantasize?

3. Rituals: Write down your Rituals. These were the activities that you did when prepping to use. Do you identify with the "high" of the ritual? How?

4. Using: What did you use and how did you use it? Was anyone else involved? Did your choices in people, substances, or situations change over time? Now pick your last or worst bout of using and describe it.

5. Despair/Shame/Guilt: Describe how you felt about yourself after that worst time. Did you break any agreements as a result of using? Did the fantasy turn out like you expected?

6. Isolation: Do you feel isolated around your using? Describe a time when you felt most isolated.

7. Do you think you have crossed the "invisible line" into addiction or compulsive behavior? Explain.

8. Share your Addiction Cycle inventory with someone with whom you feel comfortable enough. Maybe it's your therapist or another sober person. Be completely honest. Don't leave anything out. If you don't feel safe yet, find someone you think may be trustworthy, and share with them when you are ready.

9. If you finished this exercise without using, give yourself a pat on the back. This stuff can be tough to look at when you are sober. It is okay to feel good about the work you've done.

Straight Shot (5–10 Minutes)

1. Do you think you have crossed the "invisible line" into addiction or compulsive, maladaptive behavior? Explain.

2. Describe how you relate to the Addiction Cycle with your therapist or a sober friend.

Notes

1. Patrick Carnes, *Out of the Shadows: Understanding Sexual Addiction*, 3rd ed. (Center City, MN: Hazelden, 2001), 19–20. Carnes, renowned author and specialist in the treatment of sexual addiction, describes the Addiction Cycle but specific to the four stages of sexual addiction (i.e., Preoccupation, Ritualization, Sexual Compulsivity, and Despair). The Addiction Cycle in this book refers to any addiction.
2. Ronald A. Ruden and Marcia Byalick, *The Craving Brain*, 2nd ed. (New York: Harper, 2003), 1. According to Ruden and Byalick, "Gotta have it" is the driving thought of an addict, with addiction not being a "matter of will." This book goes on to explain the science that supports these ideas, with dopamine being a major player.
3. *Alcoholics Anonymous*, 4th ed. (New York: Alcoholics Anonymous World Services, 2001), xxviii and xxx. Dr. W. D. Silkworth, who was a medical doctor and specialist in treating alcoholism in the 1930s, wrote a letter in 1939 for the first edition of the Big Book, *Alcoholics Anonymous*. In this letter, Dr. Silkworth introduces the allergy idea, stating he understands alcoholism to be not a moral weakness but "the manifestation of an allergy," coupled with the mental obsession to drink. Also, for those of you unfamiliar with the Big Book (so named because of the thickness of the paper with the first printing), this is the main text for alcoholics in recovery in the Twelve Step program. Other Twelve Step programs refer to the Big Book and use their own recovery literature as well.
4. Nora D. Volkow, George F. Koob, and A. Thomas McLellan, "Neurobiologic Advances from the Brain Disease Model of Addiction," *New England Journal of Medicine* 374 (2016): 363–371, https://doi.org/10.1056/NEJMra1511480.
5. Ernest Kurtz, *Not-God: A History of Alcoholics Anonymous* (Center City, MN: Hazelden, 1991), 22.
6. Ruden and Byalick, *The Craving Brain*, 93. If you want to watch a quick synopsis of the main ideas presented in *The Craving Brain*, Google the 7-minute animated film, *The Pathology of Addiction*, by Janis Dougherty. This film makes the science part fun and entertaining.
7. Anna Lembke, *Dopamine Nation: Finding Balance in the Age of Indulgence* (New York: Dutton, 2021), 53–57. This pursuit to gratify brings us back to the physiological—repeated exposure (tolerance) to the neurotransmitter dopamine leads to anhedonia, which is the inability to enjoy pleasure of any kind. A must read, by the way.
8. "Opioid and Heroin Addiction," Hazelden Betty Ford Foundation, accessed December 19, 2021, www.hazeldenbettyford.org/addiction/types-of-addiction/opioids.
9. Carlo DiClemente, *Addiction and Change: How Addictions Develop and Addicted People Recover* (New York: The Guilford Press, 2018), 26–31. This widely used scholarly text for addiction studies presents five stages of change in the Transtheoretical Model. Three stages come before abstinence: Precontemplation, Contemplation, and Preparation (with the last two stages as Action and Maintenance).
10. Gabor Maté, *In the Realm of Hungry Ghosts: Close Encounters With Addiction* (Berkeley, CA: North Atlantic Books, 2010), 109–120.

Works Cited

Alcoholics Anonymous. *Alcoholics Anonymous: Big Book Reference Edition for Addiction Treatment*. 4th ed. New York: Alcoholics Anonymous, 2014.

Carnes, Patrick. *Out of the Shadows: Understanding Sexual Addiction*. 3rd ed. Center City, MN: Hazelden, 2001.

DiClemente, Carlo. *Addiction and Change: How Addictions Develop and Addicted People Recover.* 2nd ed. New York: The Guilford Press, 2018.

Hazelden Betty Ford Foundation. "Opioid and Heroin Addiction." Accessed December 19, 2021. www.hazeldenbettyford.org/addiction/types-of-addiction/opioids.

Kurtz, Ernest. *Not-God: A History of Alcoholics Anonymous.* Center City, MN: Hazelden, 1991.

Lembke, Anna. *Dopamine Nation: Finding Balance in the Age of Indulgence.* New York: Dutton, 2021.

Maté, Gabor. *In the Realm of Hungry Ghosts: Close Encounters With Addiction.* Berkeley, CA: North Atlantic Books, 2010.

Ruden, Ronald A., and Marcia Byalick. *The Craving Brain.* 2nd ed. New York: Harper-Collins, 2000.

Volkow, Nora D., George F. Koob, and A. Thomas McLellan. "Neurobiologic Advances from the Brain Disease Model of Addiction." *New England Journal of Medicine* 374 (2016): 363–371. https://doi.org/10.1056/NEJMra1511480.

Part Two

Freedom!

2 The Recovery Cycle

In This Chapter

- How Do I Enter the Recovery Cycle?
- Break Free
- Four Cornerstones of Transformation
- Triggers and Cravings—They Don't Magically Disappear

Are you ready to enter the Recovery Cycle? The place where recovering people can individuate, actualize, and discover how to fall in love with the sober life?

Leaving behind the addictive prison, that walled off place of illusion and doom, it's now time to step into the boundless, creative journey of recovery. A custom-designed life trip beckons, where the freedom to be you awaits!

How Do I Enter the Recovery Cycle?

I can make the answer to this question easy for you: Since you are reading this, you have entered the Recovery Cycle. Your mindset is thinking about, and focusing on, recovery. This means you have a Recovery Focus. But we are getting ahead of ourselves.

You may be thinking, *I don't get it.* Maybe your thinking is still preoccupied with your drug of choice or maybe you have a trigger that is bugging you. Perhaps there is something in you that wants to keep the door open to using or acting out again. That's fine. That's your choice. It really is your choice. No one can tell you when you are done.

So, if you aren't quite done with alcohol, acting out sexually, or whatever thing you do, you could go back to the Addiction Cycle and see how it goes. Before you do, though, think through your last bender or bout of addictive behavior. Do you want to feel that demoralization again? If not, keep reading to gather more information. If you're still reading this, however, your focus is on recovery. You are on your way to your custom-made recovery and maybe don't know it. Even if you feel hopeless, fragile, or damaged in some way, recovery can happen for you. Keep in mind:

Healing and feeling good are possible in recovery.

DOI: 10.4324/9781003293231-5

You get to heal and feel good being you in recovery. This is the Recovery Cycle's promise.

Break Free

Have you ever wanted the freedom to just be you, without your addiction? Enter the Recovery Cycle, a simple recovery plan which supports you being sober and becoming the person you want to be in your life. It is a way to break free and heal from addiction.

With the Recovery Cycle, there are no rules to follow. You will have the freedom to choose your own style of recovery. This is your life, and you get to choose how you want to live it. There is no one way to do sobriety. You are free to be YOU. **This YOU in caps is the person you have always wanted to be, without your drug (or behavior that is causing problems for you).**

The cycle is simple and supports you being in charge of how you want to live sober. If there are only two takeaways from this book, they are:

1. You have permission to be YOU
2. You have a choice in how you want to be YOU in your life

Any good mental health professional will support you being the adult you want to be.

If abstinent, you have a choice about how you can be YOU. If you are engaged in your addiction, you don't have that choice. So, if you want to stay addicted, that's up to you, but if you truly want freedom and choice in your life—if you want recovery—know that:

> **Recovery can only happen with abstinence, and abstinence means you are not engaging in your addiction.**

Bottom line? *Abstinence is necessary for recovery.* This means not even a little using or acting out compulsively.

Think of a warm cup of comforting hot chocolate and then adding some fish sauce to it. No matter how much or little you add, if even a drop, your hot chocolate is going to taste fishy. The hot chocolate with the fish sauce isn't hot chocolate anymore but something a little stinky and not quite itself. Using your drug, no matter how much or how little, is still using.

With the foundation of abstinence underscored, we are now ready for a brief look at the Recovery Cycle, your personal plan for freedom, healing, and transformation.

Four Cornerstones of Transformation

The Recovery Cycle, shown in Figure 2.1 (and in the Appendix), is the positive mirror image of the Addiction Cycle. You will see the four cornerstones of the Recovery Cycle, which are:

Recovery Cycle

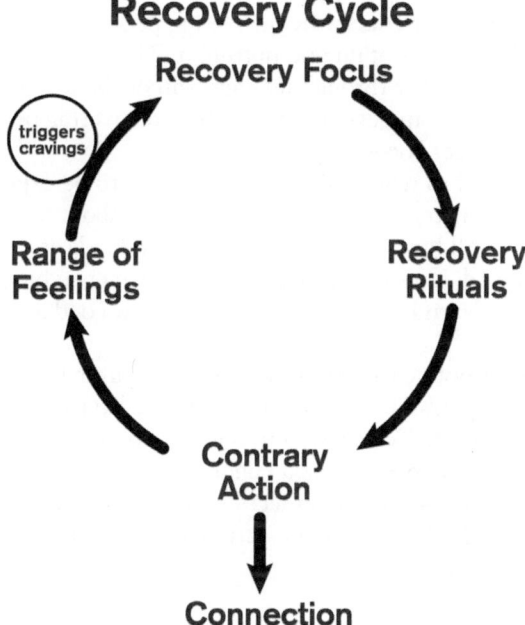

Figure 2.1 The Recovery Cycle.

1. *Recovery Focus*: A mindset focused on recovery and how to attain and maintain it. This includes a finer focus on the kind of life and relationships the recovering person wants. Also, whereas Preoccupation (in the Addiction Cycle) implies an agitated obsessiveness, Focus in recovery means attention and concentration toward the positive.

2. *Recovery Rituals*: Consistent activities and behaviors that support a recovery program. Carefully chosen Rituals are built into a successful recovery and inspire continued abstinence, consciousness about one's part in one's own recovery, and Contrary Action.

3. *Contrary Action*: Taking positive action rather than resorting to habitual, self-destructive behaviors. It is the way to break patterns that keep addicts stuck and discontented.

   Abstinence is taking Contrary Action in early recovery, but Contrary Action is also doing things differently in other areas of life as well. With Contrary Action, a host of feelings will undoubtedly surface.

4. *Range of Feelings*: Once the most basic Contrary Action is taken—meaning there has been no more engaging in the addiction—the addict's feelings are no longer isolated to guilt, shame, and despair (from the comedown after using). Instead, an expanded Range of Feelings will be experienced with all new sober experiences—and that range is wide.

Feelings, both positive and not-so-positive, are part of being human. Regardless of the emotions experienced, the recovering person's focus can shift back to recovery and how to maintain and nurture it. Think "growing pains." The satisfaction of staying sober through feelings—all of them—and feeling hope with a greater sense of connection is part of how recovering people make this shift back to a Recovery Focus.

Note: Getting used to new feelings is normal and to be expected. Feelings are what many addicts try to avoid. The main point about this feeling stuff is to expect that you will have many feelings about all kinds of things as a result of staying sober and doing some things differently. An even bigger note is that in recovery, we can learn how to experience and grow good feelings, but more on that later.

Connection: Now, notice the arrow pointing down from Contrary Action to Connection. Whereas Using in the Addiction Cycle led to Isolation, Contrary Action leads to a greater Connection to oneself, other people, and for many, something greater than oneself (i.e., a Higher Power/Universal Spirit/Mother Nature/God, etc.). This sense of Connection inspires hope and will be vital for long-term recovery. We'll discuss Connection more in Chapter 6, but for now, know this Connection feels good.

Triggers and Cravings—They Don't Magically Disappear

You will see that Triggers and Cravings are just to the left, as they were in the Addiction Cycle. Cravings may or may not go away for a while. Triggers will always be lurking here and there. It is safe to say with emphasis that:

Triggers must be dealt with consciously throughout recovery.

Dealing with triggers doesn't have to be that big of a deal, though, because with support and some recovery, triggers lose a lot of power. It's always good to remember, however, that a trigger's job is to get you to use—to hook you back into the insane confinement of the merry-go-round Addiction Cycle. The good news is that you will have many tools in your simple recovery plan that will help you deal effectively with triggers so you can stay clean, sane, and—here's the best part—even serene.

A Bit on Brokenness Before Moving On

If you've admitted you have a problem, you probably feel a little broken. Or perhaps you feel irrevocably shattered. Maybe your heart hurts and you have fractured or meaningless relationships. Or possibly everything is okay on the outside, but on the inside, you know something is awfully wrong. You might describe what you have as soul sickness. Whatever your demoralization or ache, keep in mind that this is normal for many people beginning in recovery (and maybe for some with some sober time, but I'll keep the focus for those newly sober here).

Addicts in the grip of addiction feel broken, in a sense. Wounded would be another word we could use to describe those new to recovery. Until we can admit there is something wrong with our using—that the using has caused a problem in some way—there is no chance for recovery. We must admit what is broken to fix it. Have you ever felt wounded or broken in a way?

A car mechanic doesn't work on engines that are functioning. A broken engine is brought into the mechanic's shop, and then the mechanic fixes the engine. The process to restoring a broken engine is simple:

1. Diagnose the engine's problem.
2. Fix the engine's problem.

The good news about a broken engine is that it can be restored. That said, the mechanic needs to know what a working engine looks like to repair it. If he didn't know how a functioning engine operated, or what it looked like, or how to fix it, how would he know how to repair it?

In a similar way, if an addict feels broken and doesn't have any idea of what a functioning sober life looks like and what the upkeep of this life will entail, how will he know how to fix the addiction problem and live in recovery?

If you are an addict and think your internal engine is broken, you will want to envision a functioning recovery if you want any real life-giving spark in your life. That said, keep in mind:

Although you may feel broken, YOU are not broken.

The analogy of the engine being broken is about a machine. People are not machines. Addicted people may do things that are a bit wonky, but the essence of being human is an ever-evolving state of becoming congruent with oneself as we make it through the bumps in life.

Addiction, sobering up—and just plain living—can be bumpy and messy. Feeling broken is just a part of being in the bumpy mess. *Feeling* broken, though, is not *being* broken.

As addicts who are ready to sober up, we know what broken, wounded, and heartsick feels like, but what about healing? What does healing in recovery look like? How do we heal and feel better while creating the sober life we want? The next chapter will help answer these questions.

Recovery Recap

- You have permission to be YOU, and how you want to be YOU is your choice.
- Recovery can only happen with abstinence from your drug or compulsive behavior.
- The four cornerstones of the Recovery Cycle are Recovery Focus, Recovery Rituals, Contrary Action, and Range of Feelings.
- Connection (a result of Contrary Action) is a part of recovery and feels good.
- Triggers must be dealt with consciously throughout recovery and life.
- If your heart hurts because of your addiction, or you feel hopeless or broken, healing and feeling better is possible in recovery.
- Feeling broken doesn't mean you are broken.
- Envisioning a functioning recovery is part of how you will begin to heal and feel better.

Clinician's Corner

The Recovery Cycle Inventory will help you acquire a better understanding of the recovery process—regardless of what program your client chooses for sobriety. The inventory questions will also help guide a frank talk about sobriety and help your client warm up to what to expect in recovery. Keep in mind some are slow to warm, while others have a hot readiness to do whatever it takes right away.

Remember: Many paths of recovery exist today, and any good program will encompass all elements of the Recovery Cycle.

Support your clients in whatever program they choose. Honor their choice and work with it. Discover what they like about it. Or, if something isn't working, this is where you can assist in exploring what strategies or program might work better going forward.

As you did in the last chapter and will do for each chapter, you answer the questions, too, now that you're abstinent from that thing you decided to give up as you read this book.

In session, make use of the whiteboard or oversized wall Post-It to diagram the Recovery Cycle so it is in your clients' line of sight.

Recovery Cycle Inventory (30–60 Minutes)

Review the Recovery Cycle (Figure 2.1) and write out your answers.

1. Recovery Focus: What thoughts do you have about your sobriety and your program (if you belong to one)?

    If not in a program, what are your reasons for not connecting with one? Do you have any judgments or fear? Explain.

    If new to sobriety, what thoughts do you have about abstinence? What do you think you will need to do to stay sober? What do you want to do to stay sober?

    Who will be your guide? If you don't know, do you have someone in mind? What do you want or expect in a sober guide?

    Other thoughts that may come up for you may be about literature, meetings, and relationships. Describe any thoughts about these or anything else.

2. Recovery Rituals: List any sober Recovery Rituals you have now or any you want to incorporate into your recovery program.

    Do your Rituals speak to you personally? How do you know this?

3. Contrary Action: What is your understanding of Contrary Action?

    List any positive actions you have taken while sober. Maybe these actions were out of your comfort zone. This could be anything from walking away from a potential fistfight when feeling provoked (perhaps you used to fight anytime you felt angry) to making your bed in the morning (maybe you never made your bed) to structuring your evening time around sober meetings and family time (instead of using/acting out).

4. Range of Feelings: What is your comfort level with discussing feelings, on a scale from 1 to 10 (10 being most uncomfortable)? Do you notice your feelings? Can you recall the feelings you had the last time you used or acted out?

    Now sober, can you describe what it feels like to choose sobriety (instead of using)?

    List any feelings you have had as a result of staying abstinent and taking Contrary Action (e.g., "I felt kind of angry not getting into a fist fight with that guy, but after felt proud of myself that I didn't engage and end up in jail").

5. Connection: Describe a time when you felt most connected in a positive way. This could be when you were a child or a time more recent in sobriety. Were you with someone/others/alone? Where were you? What were you doing?

6. If you've completed this exercise, congratulations! It is not always easy to sit and do the work of recovery, so, give yourself a pat on the back.

Straight Shot (5–10 Minutes)

1. How do you understand the Recovery Cycle?
2. Plug yourself into each cornerstone of the Recovery Cycle. Describe how you relate or don't. Share your findings with your therapist or sober friend.

3 Define Your Recovery, Design Your Life

In This Chapter

- What Is a Recovery Focus?
- What About a Relationship Focus?
- Any Way You Want It
- Bottoms Up or Choice

With good focus comes definition. We are about to home in on just exactly how to aim the recovering person's mindset toward a better quality of thought and, therefore, a higher quality of life. A good and steady Recovery Focus will define the sober person's abstinence and new drug-free life. Giving up the addiction is only the beginning.

What Is a Recovery Focus?

As said in the last chapter, a Recovery Focus, the first cornerstone of the Recovery Cycle, is not the obsessive, distracting-from-your-life Preoccupation of the Addiction Cycle. **A Recovery Focus is the positive attention and concentration you direct toward abstinence and your life in recovery**. Another way of saying this is: The recovering person's mindset is focused on recovery and how to attain and maintain it.

Maintaining Focus on abstinence—and staying abstinent—is the beginning of physical sobriety. A healthy recovery includes emotional sobriety, as well (which, in brief, means the ability to accept and regulate one's feelings and act in a healthy way). So, to develop the kind of relationships and life the recovering person wants will include a Focus beyond just staying abstinent.

So, what does this mean?

When you focus on something, you need to know what your target of focus looks like if you want to hit the bullseye. If you don't know what your recovery—the target—looks like, how will you know where to aim your focus? The point of this chapter is to know what you want your recovery to look like so you can focus on it.

If you're anything like I was in early recovery, you are thinking about sobriety a lot. You may be thinking about what it will take to stay sober and what you

DOI: 10.4324/9781003293231-6

will have to do. You might be thinking recovery is attainable and valuable. You might think about going to the liquor store, but don't, because you are meeting up with a sober friend instead. You find yourself thinking about how you will tell your friend that you stayed sober that day.

All these thoughts contribute to a good focus on abstinence—which, again, is the beginning of any recovery. But there is more to recovery than just quitting the drug (which we know, though, is the essential requirement for recovery). After the post-sobriety hoopla has died down and we have a little time in sobriety, there is the business of everyday living that is bound to get in the way of all good intentions to stay sober.

Everyday Living Example in Sobriety

(Hint: Have you ever heard of the acronym ANTS?)

7:00 A.M.

Your alarm goes off. It seems like a personal hell has broken loose in your head. You are irritated that you must go into work. You think your co-worker is lazy. You don't like him. *My boss is not that great either*, you think. Then you wonder why your girlfriend said what she said to you last night, and you decide you won't call her for a week, even though you typically talk every day. You ruminate about how she could be so insensitive. *Yah*, you decide, *I'll definitely make her pay*. Suddenly, your cat, Whiskers, jumps on the bed and is meowing like crazy. You are annoyed—no, mad—because Whiskers interrupted your train of thinking about what you would say to your girlfriend next week. You reluctantly get up and tell your annoying feline to leave you alone.

On your way to the shower, you remember something irritating your sister said. While showering, your thoughts bat around from *girlfriend* to *lazy co-worker*, to *jerk boss* to *why did I get a cat?*

As you wash your hair you think, *My mom didn't do that good of a job, it's no wonder I'm not that great and my sister is so weird. My friends really aren't that great either, and why does everyone want something from me? People are overrated. I'm better off alone.*

Out of the shower, drying off, you think, *I'm such a downer, why was I born anyway? I think I'll call in sick. Then I won't have to deal with anyone. Maybe I'll take a sleeping pill.* Then you glance at the clock.

7:13 A.M.

You've been awake not quite 15 minutes. Then Whiskers meows at your feet—again—wanting to be fed.

Does this sound like Another Negative Thought Syndrome, a.k.a. ANTS?

This might not be exactly how your brain thinks on any day, but the point is when the addict brain is without right focus, it can go willy-nilly in a very bad way. Every day can become a chore where we find others annoying and ourselves not so great either. Let's face it. If everything was hunky-dory in our thinking, we might not have turned to our addictions in the first place.

Sorting out squirrely thinking and getting perspective can surprisingly change a bad day into a good one and can support better relationships in recovery, too. If anything or anyone is bugging you, do the Get it Out on Paper! writing exercise. Writing is a way to get stuff out of you and will be a valuable addition to your recovery tool kit.

Get It Out on Paper!

1. Take 15–20 minutes to write about anything or anyone that is annoying you. Don't edit yourself or worry about spelling, punctuation, or grammar. Just write. This exercise is not about pretending you feel better than you do or that you are a good person. It is about getting every last bit out on paper, no matter how ugly. Keep what you wrote in a safe place until the next day. No need to share this with anyone.
2. The next day, read what you wrote out loud to yourself, as if your friend wrote it and is now reading it to you.

What did you notice after reading your writing out loud? Is there a difference between how you felt between the first and second days? What is the difference?

What About a Relationship Focus?

The addictions of our choosing kept us isolated and most likely in dysfunctional or obsession-riddled relationships. Then, when we sober up, we still have problems in our relationships. These problems stem from how we think about our relationships—and everything else, too. It is how we think that causes many of our problems. Our difficulties often lie in our perceptions. Like in the example earlier, we might end up thinking how we can deal with people rather than relate to them in a caring way. Would you rather be dealt with or related to?

Relationships in Recovery

Relationships become a major focus of attention in recovery. This focus can take a downturn into negative, obsessive, and dysfunctional thinking. This kind of focus, with an old, scratched lens, can threaten sobriety.

Developing healthy and caring relationships (with ourselves and others) not only helps keep us sober but also makes recovery—and life—meaningful and worth the effort. It is true for many sober people that:

A big part of recovery includes cultivating healthy and caring relationships.

The idea of defining your own recovery with the goal of functioning in more healthy and caring relationships is a good one.[1] Keeping a focus on relationships in a fixated, obsessive (i.e., preoccupied) way is not the idea though!

For any recovery to take hold, we must wrangle our thinking and aim it toward recovery. Defining what recovery means for you may be a challenge. How you define your recovery is up to you. I suggest, though, that you **consider cultivating healthy caring relationships as part of how you define your recovery**. This means envisioning and developing positive relationships with others, as well as a positive relationship with yourself, and your selves. Yes, that's right. Your *selves*.

The Committee

After sobering up, you may notice a committee lives in your head. My personal favorites are the critic, the case-builder, and the victim. Sometimes the self-righteous one rears up, too. You may have your own special darlings. (Think about that one troublesome family member at holiday gatherings or celebrations and imagine him or her living in your head.) I mentioned the more obnoxious examples because they seem to be the ones who cause so much trouble within ourselves and in our relationships.

In recovery, it is our responsibility to find a positive way to relate to these offensive members and not let them derail good focus. When we don't let these unruly members take over our thinking, we can have right focus and a good life. (And better holidays and family gatherings too.)

In early recovery, my committee members were the prime manufacturers of misery and gloom. I didn't realize there was an off-key chorus in my head, I just knew I didn't feel good. Many mornings I would wake up feeling, well, just wrong. I needed a big shift in perspective each day for quite a while.

My Recovery Focus included believing that recovery included feeling good (even on days when I didn't) and that I was worthy of being alive. This perspective is still one I hold dear, especially on those evenings when the voices chime in telling me, *It's no use*, or, *You aren't that smart*, or *They are all going to snicker behind your back*.

In whatever we do in recovery—in life—we are there and so are people. People and voices seem to be everywhere, unless you are a complete recluse. But even alone on some deserted island or in outer space, there will be the voices in our heads. How we think about people and ourselves has been such a big problem for so many addicted people that **it makes sense to define part** of recovery as being in right relationship with ourselves and others. That said, you still get to define recovery how you want. Just be aware that healthy, caring relationships are vital to a solid recovery. Ultimately, you create the life and relationships you want.

Any Way You Want It

That's right. Your recovery can be any way you want it.

It can't be overstated that it is up to you to define your idea of recovery. How you define it is all your choice. Whether you have a positive attitude or negative outlook is all up to you. You get this choice when you are abstinent. For me, some days it takes work to switch my perspective so I can have a good day (and a good life).

Ideally, your idea of recovery is positive for you. You get to define your recovery any way you want because you get to be YOU.

When you define your recovery, you design your life.

Think about that statement a minute.

If I'm defining my recovery as something worthwhile, where I feel connected to myself and others in positive way, then I'm designing how I want my life and relationships to be. Then, I can live my recovery mindset in all I do—it goes with me everywhere. At home, at work, at play, and on elevators and freeways in between, too. In other words, my recovery is my life. I have the choice to define my recovery as drudgery and separate from the rest of my life, sure, but then I'll be living a downer recovery; how could that not carry into the rest of my life?

Keeping a positive Focus can turn a perceived down-in-the dumps moment into a focused, elevated one. And enough higher moments can add up to the good sober life you want.

Consider these comments from newly sober people about how they keep a Recovery Focus and move their lives in a direction they want.

- "When I start feeling that old familiar hopeless feeling, I do my best to switch my thinking into being grateful that I'm not hung over, and then I call someone who is in recovery."
- "Because I haven't acted out, I am beginning to see what triggers me. I used to think something was wrong with me and that I had no choice. Now I know I have a choice in everything. Before recovery, I didn't know I had a choice in much."
- "I'm doing some thinking about what kind of marriage I want in recovery, and how I can earn the trust of my family back."
- "In rehab we discussed how to get through the holidays sober, and I designed a plan for myself with my counselor."
- "I listen to what my sponsor tells me. I never used to listen to anyone. I'm learning to be more open, and this is how I want to be in my life in general."

- "My sober friends and I get together and laugh a lot about how we are recovering in our program. In a fun way, we hold each other accountable for our sobriety. I've always wanted friendships like this."
- "Part of my Recovery Focus is visualizing how I can be light and polite to people, especially my boss. She really gets my goat, but I want to be a respectful employee in my recovery."
- "I think about how recovery will be a big change in my life. I am a little scared, but willing to do anything to get my self-respect back. I don't know exactly what is ahead, but my plan is to stick with others who are comfortable in their recovery."

If you have had any thoughts remotely like any of these you have had a Recovery Focus for at least a part of the time. The idea is to build on this mindset. The prize of this focus is a better life. The life you've envisioned and decided you want.

In case you didn't notice, in the previous list of thoughts the people were not thinking about how to get their drug. Nor were they fantasizing about the past and rationalizing, "It wasn't that bad." One big trap for addicts is to forget there was a problem, which leads back to using. It's as if part of the brain has gone to sleep while driving and there is an automatic turn down Addiction Street.

Do You Want to Connect to Your Soul?

Let's face it, if you're not focused on recovery, you are bound to use again, and, using only leads to bad feelings, problems, and a feeling you might call soul sickness. Your soul is not sick, however. You might have just numbed yourself to the point where it is so far away you can't connect with it. **This soul sickness, which really is a soul disconnect, is a deeply rooted, aching feeling that you are incongruent with your innermost self in some profound way, perhaps acting in ways that are not you.**

This disparity comes with an awful-feeling combo of hopelessness, helplessness, and a gripping despondency. This is the neighborhood of Addiction Street.

With no thought of recovery when you were using, could you manage to stay sober and connected to your innermost self? My bet is no, or you wouldn't be reading this book. So, good for you that you are here now, focused on recovery. By focusing, in the way this book describes, you can stay on the road of recovery and connect back to YOU.

Want More Good Reasons for a Recovery Focus?

From my own experience and working with others, I've come up with what I think are some good reasons for a Recovery Focus. See if these reasons make any sense to you.

- **The greater the Recovery Focus, the greater the chances of avoiding the rituals of using.** This means your chances are better for establishing rituals and practices which support a drug-free life. And a drug-free life includes good feelings and joy. This is an important point to remember (and significant prize) no matter how long you are sober.

- **A sustained Recovery Focus will root in your psyche the recovery—and life—you want for yourself.** Your recovery, *as you define it*, will have personal meaning to you and will need attention, thought, and care. Your chances of staying sober long-term are increased when your brain is trained to care about your recovery, to the point where it is almost automatic.

- **A Recovery Focus, defined in your own positive way, can help you avoid the downward spiral of negative thinking.** Addicts prone to the pitfalls of negative, obsessive, or self-destructive thinking will do better and feel better when they think better. Having no mind-point toward recovery is in a sense normal for addicts, though.

Our mental state has been habituated to focusing on and procuring the drug of choice and then using it (often to avoid something). In a way, an addict's normal state is to be drunk, whether drunk on booze, drunk at a casino, or drunk with whatever drug or behavior tweaks our beak for that minute. Using makes us feel normal. After sobering up, though, our normal is often imbued with negative thinking.

This negative thinking produces not-so-great feelings, and the not-so-great feelings, in turn, reinforce the negative thinking. With this, there is a rumination feedback loop. This loop, whether we like to admit it or not, often becomes our new normal, unless we do something different with our thinking. **With good Focus—rerouting our thinking in a positive direction—we forge a new state of normal. This new state includes good feelings and joy.**

For many, this recovery way of thinking may trigger you to feel a little uncomfortable or scared, because, in a sense, it is abnormal for you. This is all (not to overuse the word but here it goes) normal. If you are confused, don't try to figure it out. Just remember:

Your Recovery Focus will be a new way to aim your brain.

Maintaining this aim will help you build the solid recovery—and life—you want.

Recovery is kind of like learning to drive. There will be learning curves on the road for sure, but with consistent practice, it becomes easier and semi-automatic. On our journey, though, we need to stay awake and conscious with our eyes open if we want to enjoy the trip and avoid the route to Addiction Street. What turn are you taking right now?

Want Out of Scary Neighborhoods?

If (or for some of us, when) your brain takes a turn for the worse and ends up in a dark, scary, or freaky neighborhood, not to worry. You can leave

Addiction Street and get your brain back on track. Here are some ideas to help you jumpstart your way back to Recovery Road where your soul can feel most nurtured.

1. **Identify who you want to support you in your sober journey.** You will need support. Addicts have difficulty staying sober without it. In Twelve Step programs, there is a tremendous amount of support from experts. These experts, as I mean it, are the ones who are successfully living drug free or abstaining from acting out. They know addiction firsthand and understand. Other programs are out there, too, and digital offerings abound. I suggest, though, meeting in person. Sober face-to-face experience is invaluable.

    Mental health professionals, too, can be of great support, but the experts— the addicts like yourself—are the ones who will be your staple.

2. **Contact your support person (the guide you identified in the last chapter) or a sober friend.** Tell this person about your desire to stay sober or share what's going on in your head.

3. **Read recovery literature.** This may help you decide if you want to go to a Twelve Step program or try another way to get support. The Twelve Step programs (a massive study shows) offer success that is hard to deny.[2] There are many pamphlets and books available from Twelve Step and other programs that have tons of information. Scores of meditation/daily readers are available as well.

4. **Get to know your triggers, but don't pull the trigger.** Triggers, as discussed earlier, are guaranteed in recovery. Those who stay sober talk to others about their triggers and share with each other what to do— instead of pulling the trigger.

    Remember: Triggers can be thoughts, feelings, people, places, and things—basically, anything that sends the brain down the path of thinking about using. Negative thinking, a.k.a. "stinking thinking," is a big trigger for a lot of sober people. It's a good idea to share negative thinking with other recovering people.

5. **Google a Twelve Step group specific to your addiction.** Find the meeting directory for your area. See where the meetings are and make a plan to go. (Then, go.)

6. **Check out other support groups.** Today, a plethora of sober support exists, especially for those who have a problem with alcohol. Get online and do your research. I actually know someone who uses Instagram for their sober support.

These are just some of the ways you can recharge your brain back to a Recovery Focus.

Too Much Focus?

Perhaps you think this is all too much focusing on recovery.

It's true. Some recovering people are preoccupied with sobriety to the point of hyper obsession. Having an obsessive approach to recovery is not necessarily a bad thing, though.

If anyone has a judgment about being passionately consumed with recovery, that's your right, but think about it a minute. If Bill Wilson, cofounder of Alcoholics Anonymous, hadn't been fanatical about his own recovery, the program of AA wouldn't be around today. And, because of the successful, widely used Twelve Step program of AA, there are now programs for almost any addiction. Many people are living successful, dynamic lives without their drug because of this one man's fervent focus. Keep in mind, however, that sometimes an obsessive focus on the program, for some, can become a secondary addiction.

Bottoms Up or Choice

Some say that addicts in the clutches of their addiction don't have a choice about using. They feel doomed and sentenced to their life of addiction. The Big Book of Alcoholics Anonymous sums up the concept in this way:

> The fact is that most alcoholics, for reasons yet obscure, have lost the power of choice in drink. Our so called will power becomes practically nonexistent. We are unable, at certain times, to bring to our consciousness with sufficient force the memory of even a week or month ago. We are without defense against the first drink.[3]

Remember, the drink, as stated in the previous paragraph and as I mean it, is that something personal to you: gambling, porn, pills, sugar, or anything else. All addictions involve the reward system in the brain in a similar way, which energizes the compulsion.[4]

I've certainly experienced this lack of choice. Have you? Take a few minutes to think about the moment before you used the last time. Was it possible to have a Recovery Focus? Did you really have a choice? If you are like most addicts, you probably felt you didn't have a choice. (In a way, the prefrontal cortex gets hijacked by the pleasure center.)

At some point, though, addicts may come to experience that they do have a choice.

I had a choice the day I hit my own personal bottom. My bottom was light-weight compared to other bottoms I've heard about.

After many attempts to stop drinking and using cocaine, and one botched suicide attempt which was really a cry for help, one night I decided I wanted to do heroin, drive off a cliff into the ocean, and kill myself. A former heroin addict, someone I had met in rehab the previous month who was barely sober himself, wouldn't go along with my brilliant plan. He wouldn't get me the heroin. I'll always be grateful for that. He looked at me with such pity—I'll never forget that look.

The next morning that same heroin addict and my mother escorted me back to the same rehab I had left a few weeks earlier. It was a month before my 21st birthday. On that day I just knew deep down the jig was up. My reasoning was that if I did heroin, I would probably kill myself, and I didn't want to die. I felt frightened and desperate. I'd felt this way before, but this time, for whatever reason, I had a choice.

High, Low, Soft, and Hard—Bottoms Are Different

Every addict's bottom is different. Driving drunk with kids in the car, felony drunk driving, jail time, losing a job, embarrassing oneself at a funeral (I know someone who danced topless on a table at a funeral), getting caught in an online affair, gaining 300 pounds—these might all be things that get the addict to choose sobriety, or maybe not. This is part of the mystery about when an addict gets sober—each addict's bottom is personal. Often, outside circumstances just don't have much to do with the reason an addict chooses to get sober. The key point is:

> **When someone hits their personal bottom, something incredible**
> **happens that starts them on their journey to recovery:**
> **a psychic shift.**

The Psychic Shift

The most mysterious element about choice and hitting bottom is the experience of the psychic shift:

> Once a psychic change has occurred, the very same person who seemed doomed, who had so many problems he despaired of ever solving them, suddenly finds himself easily able to control his desire for alcohol, the only effort necessary being that required to follow a few simple rules.[5]

You probably noticed in the aforementioned statement about following "a few simple rules." Not to worry if you aren't a rule follower. Just think of having an open mind to do some things differently—with the prize of being "easily able" to control your desire for your drug. One thing we can do differently is keep a Recovery Focus. This is a surprisingly simple thing to do once we've had the necessary shift in thinking—once we realize we can make a choice. This goes for alcohol or anything else.

Why any one of us gets and stays sober is a huge mystery. Again, our natural state as addicts seems to be that of being drunk or wanting to get drunk (or act out compulsively). There is good news, though. You can be one of the sober ones, too. You can have the recovery you want. With abstinence and your personal realization that you are done using, you will have a choice.

Once addicts can make the choice to stay abstinent, they can focus on recovery and begin their new drug-free life.

I want to add a note here about opioid addiction, as the withdrawal and sobering up from this type of substance appears to have a different intensity than for any other kind of addiction or compulsive behavior.

With addictive opioid use, there may be a strong desire to get sober, but keeping the sober focus may prove much more challenging (according to clinicians I've spoken to in the field). Watch the series *Dopesick*, and you'll see what I mean.

First, there are the ferocious cravings from the hellacious physical withdrawal. Then, in early recovery, from what I gather after talking to a few sober opioid addicts, nothing in real life can compare to the promise of the euphoric, off-the-charts pleasure of the opioid. Someone I know said her addiction was like "being held in the arms of God, until it wasn't."

After prolonged use of opioids, the pleasure center in the brain generates a demonic pain. And opioid recovery people, like many addicts, seem to have a built-in forgetter in their brain. They forget that using ultimately causes more and more negative consequences and agonizing pain.

This forgetting mechanism, whether it can be explained by science or not, is a real thing in the mind and body of an addict, which is why so many do best with repeated reminders that ingesting the substance (or doing that compulsive behavior) isn't a pleasurable, good activity and will cause pain in the most awful way. Addicts find reminders (such as going to meetings with newly sober people) helpful well into long-term sobriety.

So, back to the point about focus: We need to keep our eye on the *real* pleasurable prizes of recovery if we want a solid, satisfying life in sobriety. The Recovery Cycle shows addicts—including opioid users—how to do just that. The idea is to increase healthy pleasure in our lives and our capacity to enjoy it. This means placing a Recovery Focus on discovering sober, healthy pleasure. Neuropsychologist Rick Hanson says, "Your attention is like a combination spotlight and vacuum cleaner: It highlights what it lands on and then sucks it into your brain—for better or worse."[6] We'll delve more into how to put the spotlight on good feelings with focused attention in Chapter 7.

To wrap up, if you are not done using, any diagram or program or all the information and focus in the world won't keep you sober. In a split second, the subconscious mind can rationalize why using is a good idea despite all worthy information and previous evidence to the contrary. The compulsion to act out addictively can defy all good reason and sound intention.

If you are having difficulty getting sober and are baffled by this, gathering the info may still be beneficial. Don't give up. There may come a day when you know there is a place where you can feel safe, understood, and free from the grip of your drug or compulsion. You can make a choice that makes good sense. With consistent effort and willingness, a Recovery Focus that works for you will come.

Recovery Recap

- A Recovery Focus is the positive attention and concentration given toward one's abstinence and life in recovery.
- Negative thinking, left untamed, will cause problems.
- Functioning in healthy, caring relationships is vital for recovery.
- Recovery is not only about abstinence but also about defining the recovery and life you want for yourself.
- Your Recovery Focus will be personal to you.
- Aiming your brain in a positive direction will keep it out of scary neighborhoods.
- Every addict's bottom is different and not necessarily determined by outside circumstances.
- Most addicts have a choice about recovery when they have had a profound shift in thinking, along with a willingness to do some things differently.
- Information alone won't keep you sober but continue to gather information—with consistent effort and willingness, your Recovery Focus will come.

Clinician's Corner

This is a great time to introduce a few minutes of quiet time with your client. Start each session with 1–5 minutes of sitting quietly, with eyes closed. The idea is for transitioning and centering. Use a timer with a gentle ring, a meditation bell, or a singing bowl.

If you have a guided meditation you like, okay, but leave at least 1 minute for quiet. Ideally your guided meditation focuses on tuning into one's heart. Our child's heart within is the best knower of our own authentic wants and dreams.

You do the exercise first on your own, as usual. You are the guide. Best to know what your client might experience on their journey so you can lead the way safely.

Minding Recovery Road (20–60 Minutes)

1. Take 1–5 minutes of quiet time (i.e., meditation), with eyes closed, before proceeding with Steps 2 and 3. This is a time to transition from the outside world into the internal world of you and your heart.

2. Define what recovery is for you. This will become increasingly important the longer you stay sober. Think about your relationships, your health, your spiritual life, your work, etc.—basically, every aspect of your life and how you want to be a sober you in it. Here are some questions to help you focus:

   • If you are in a Twelve Step program, how do you understand the steps and spirituality? If you are in another program, what stands out to you as the most important element for your sobriety? What works for you?

   • What are your reasons for wanting to be in recovery? What are the upsides to living a clean and sober life?

   • What does the sober life you want look like? What would you be doing or not doing? How are you willing to work toward this?

   • What do you think about cultivating healthy relationships as being vital to a sound recovery? Explain.

   • Do you want good communication with your friends and loved ones? What would that look/sound like? What would you be doing or not doing to get it?

   • Do you want to feel better in your body in some way and have better physical health? If yes, how would you do this?

3. Consider your heart's desires. If there is anything coming to your mind now, write it down. Maybe think of the kind of person you want to be or anything you want to do in your life.

Feel free to share your writing with your sober guide, counselor, therapist, or someone you feel safe with. Or, don't share. Whatever is comfortable for you.

Straight Shot (5–15 Minutes)

1. Sit with eyes closed for 1–5 minutes of quiet time (i.e., meditation).

2. Do you think you have hit your bottom and had any profound shift in thinking about your using or acting out? Describe.
3. Give two examples of how you keep your Recovery Focus.
4. Write out what is valuable to you about living sober.
5. What do you want most in your sober life?

Notes

1. Earnie Larsen, *Stage II Recovery: Life Beyond Addiction* (New York: HarperCollins, 1985), 11–17. Larsen makes a distinction between Stage I and Stage II Recovery: Stage I Recovery is about abstinence from the primary addiction, whereas Stage II Recovery is about how the addict defines recovery for himself with the goal of functioning more capably in healthy, caring relationships.
2. "An Update on the Evidence for Alcoholics Anonymous Participation," Recovery Research Institute, accessed December 20, 2021, www.recoveryanswers.org/research-post/update-evidence-alcoholics-anonymous-participation/. "This recently released comprehensive report systematically reviews the science to date on AA and used rigorous meta-analytic techniques to weigh the evidence" (para. 1). This review found that AA produces rates of abstinence in the short-term comparable to interventions (like Cognitive Behavioral Therapy) and outperforms them over the long-term.
3. *Alcoholics Anonymous*, 4th ed. (New York: Alcoholics Anonymous World Services, 2001), 24. This baffling lack of choice is described in detail in the chapter, "There Is a Solution." Also discussed in this chapter is a solution to recovery from alcoholism.
4. Jon E. Grant, Marc N. Potenza, Aviv Weinstein, and David A. Gorelick, "Introduction to Behavioral Addictions," *The American Journal of Drug and Alcohol Abuse* 36, no. 5 (2010): 233–241, https://doi.org/10.3109/00952990.2010.491884.
5. *Alcoholics Anonymous*, xxix. For more on the psychic shift, you will find a short description of different types of spiritual experiences in Appendix II, "Spiritual Experiences," of the Big Book, *Alcoholics Anonymous*, 567. People in recovery describe relating to the different types of spiritual experiences as described in this reading.
6. Rick Hanson, *Hardwiring Happiness: The New Brain Science of Contentment, Calm and Confidence* (New York: Random House, 2013), 11.

Works Cited

Alcoholics Anonymous. *Alcoholics Anonymous: Big Book Reference Edition for Addiction Treatment.* 4th ed. New York: Alcoholics Anonymous, 2014.

Grant, Jon E., Marc N. Potenza, Aviv Weinstein, and David A. Gorelick. "Introduction to Behavioral Addictions." *The American Journal of Drug and Alcohol Abuse* 36, no. 5 (2010): 233–241. https://doi.org/10.3109/00952990.2010.491884.

Hanson, Rick. *Hardwiring Happiness: The New Brain Science of Contentment, Calm and Confidence.* New York: Random House, 2013.

Larsen, Earnie. *Stage II Recovery: Life Beyond Addiction.* New York: HarperCollins, 1985.

Recovery Research Institute. "An Update on the Evidence for Alcoholics Anonymous Participation." Accessed December 20, 2021. www.recoveryanswers.org/research-post/update-evidence-alcoholics-anonymous-participation/.

4 Rituals That Make Good Sense

In This Chapter

- What Are Recovery Rituals?
- Are Recovery Rituals Really That Important?
- Meaning
- Rituals Made Easy

Recovery Rituals, the second cornerstone of the Recovery Cycle, are paramount for establishing a solid foundation for a custom-built sober life. Recovery Rituals that make good sense—and with personal meaning—will carry the recovering person through both good times and difficult times.

What Are Recovery Rituals?

Recovery Rituals are consistent activities that support a recovery program meaningful to you, the recovering person. Rituals are deliberately chosen and replace the rituals of using.

Now let's break these words down to bite-sized, digestible pieces:

Consistent means acting or doing something with regularity over time.
Activities are things you do.
A *recovery program* is a blueprint or plan for staying sober that includes other sober people.
Meaningful means something has purpose, is important, or has value—to YOU.
Deliberate means carefully considered and intentional.

Rituals, again, are the activities of YOUR choosing that will support the recovery YOU want. Any suggestions made in this book serve as suggestions and are not about religion, dogma, rules, regulations, or anything of the like that might spike your spine. You select and do the Recovery Rituals that work for you.

Note: If you bristle or groan at the word *rituals*, just remember you had rituals when you were using!

DOI: 10.4324/9781003293231-7

An example of a Recovery Ritual is going to a regular recovery-related meeting or calling a sober friend consistently. Another might be reading recovery literature. If these are some of your rituals, you have carefully considered and chosen them because they help you stay sober and feel better. **Whatever ritual practice you do, be conscious of its purpose, value, and importance in your life.** Also, note that *rituals* and *activities* are both plural, so this means more than one.

Are Recovery Rituals Really That Important?

The short answer? Yes. Recovery Rituals are important. Here are some reasons why.

Recovery Rituals:

- **Lead to continued abstinence**. With Recovery Rituals, a tide of support moves us toward staying abstinent, which is the most important and basic constituent of any recovery. This support comes in the form of sober people who echo the message and experience of recovery, often in mutual-help groups. Recovering people have identified many aspects of these groups as important, such as self-confidence building, developing coping skills, giving back, bonding with others in the group, and developing a sober lifestyle.[1]
- **Have meaning and value because you've chosen them**. Some people do things ritually and don't even know why they are doing them. Have you ever done a ritual (recovery-related or not) that had no meaning for you? What was it like for you? What about a ritual that had meaning for you? What was that like?

  It is important for anyone to have a choice about what they want and don't want. If you are deliberate and thoughtful about the Recovery Rituals YOU want, your engagement in them will have more meaning and value. Also, you will be more consistent in keeping the rituals.

- **Promote satisfaction and good feelings**. Doing something that has meaning with other like-minded people is an easy way to produce satisfaction and good feelings. For addicts, feeling good may be elusive, so doing something regularly where good feelings are likely seems like a no-brainer.
- **Provide consistency and structure**. For a lot of us, addictive rituals (and using) produced chaos and ultimately a lot of bad feelings, including anxiety and shame. When growing up or while using, perhaps nothing was predictable. Recovery Rituals, one part of a good sober foundation, yield stability where maybe there once was none.
- **Inspire a be-in-the-life-you-want vibe**. Your Recovery Rituals, if you've chosen well, will encourage you to engage in new, positive behaviors

which support you being YOU. You don't have to check out of your life anymore. Basically, your carefully chosen rituals present an opportunity to be truly present in your own life and in the lives of others.

- **Become the gateway for good habits**. Doing something consistently is good training for doing *more* things consistently. We do Recovery Rituals with consistency, which is the same way we develop good habits.
- **Act as a spiritual infusion**. Shared rituals bind addicts together in spirit. Going to a regular Twelve Step meeting, for example, is not a religious activity or about dogma. (You may meet some dogmatic folk in any program, by the way, so find the people and program you like.) The point is, find the group and people which foster your spirit.

Spirit, in how I mean it, is **the nonphysical, unseen (but felt) part of you that animates your being and influences your will**.

When we do Recovery Rituals together, we share energy and spirit. With this, your spirit can finally be free and congruent in this world with others—all without using your drug or compulsive behavior.

Meaning

It can't be stressed enough that sober rituals must have meaning for you. Just as you define your own recovery and what that means to you, a Recovery Ritual will support your recovery best if it speaks to you on a deep and personal level. Even if the ritual doesn't feel particularly deep, be aware of what you are getting out of it and how it is supporting the recovery you want for yourself. With this, you will be less apt to be bored or to think of rituals as rigid acts of detention and confinement. Rituals of your choosing are part of your investment in recovery and living the life you want.

Recovery is not a lifetime where you must do things you don't want to do. Anything you do is your choice. It makes sense, then, to choose rituals you want. Maybe you like to laugh, and you find a recovery meeting where people are laughing. Perhaps that's exactly what you need. I don't know anyone who could use less laughter in their life. Or maybe you like serious one-on-one discussions about the meaning of life, and you have found someone in recovery who likes that too. Perhaps the two of you meet for coffee once a week after your recovery meeting. Maybe you will discover the meaning of life in one of those conversations.

Without a recovery plan that includes Recovery Rituals as defined in this chapter, addicts can become disheartened in their loneliness and isolation without even knowing it. Some find themselves so stuck in fear and twisted thinking that it may seem difficult to find even one Recovery Ritual that feels good. Still, with being consistent, over time, eventually good feelings (and the importance, value, and purpose of your life) will come. Keep in mind that without rituals in recovery and the vital support they provide, we could end up drunk once again, acting out in a way we don't want, or just plain miserable.

Robert—A Life Without Recovery Rituals

Robert, an alcoholic who has been through more than a few rehabs, is an example of what can happen when addicts shun Recovery Rituals.

Robert started drinking in his teens. Over the years he's gotten sober many times. He's been in Twelve Step rehabs and a few Christian recovery homes. Each time Robert got sober, he maintained a certain distance from people and any ritual, unless it was something he had to do as a requirement of the program he was in at the time. With this self-imposed distance, Robert made up his mind about people and Rituals, making judgments and criticizing them in his own mind. You see, Robert grew up in a home where people were never sources of love; his self-esteem was so low that he could never allow anyone to support him. His brain created a life script about himself and people that were fervent yet false but powerfully true to him.[2] With his destiny already written by his own twisted thinking, he would act out in ways that were shockingly self-destructive. Because he could not, or would not, surrender to exposing himself to any consistency with Rituals, Robert—now 50 years later—remains for the most part isolated, intermittently addicted to pills, and disabled physically and mentally. Although abstinent for stints at a time in various rehabs, Robert has never felt the joy of being a free Robert in recovery. Without Recovery Rituals, Robert cannot, by himself, rewrite his life script. Addiction is that powerful when it runs the addict brain alone.

Are There Any Substitutes for Rituals?

The answer to this question is no. A 30-day stint at rehab won't guarantee a sound recovery, nor will reading this book or any pamphlet. And there is no miracle drug that cures addiction or heals all wounds from the past. There is just no substitute for adopting Recovery Rituals.

The consistency part, too, is just as important as the meaning part. If you have any judgment about doing something regularly for your recovery, or the idea makes you uncomfortable in any way, that's okay. Starting anything new can be strangely uncomfortable.

The concept of Acting-As-If, developed by the Austrian physician-turned-psychoanalyst Alfred Adler, might be helpful to consider as you go about doing your rituals, particularly if you are finding it difficult to participate and be consistent.

Acting-As-If

Recovery Rituals may feel forced in the beginning or feel uncomfortable in some way. This is normal for some people. Remember: **Your recovery is a new way of life and you will be doing new things to support the life YOU want.**

Doing anything new is not always comfortable. That's okay because:

Acting-As-If you are comfortable is one way to feel comfortable.

If you Act-As-If enough times, you might find yourself not only comfortable but also enjoying that which used to be uncomfortable. Keep in mind you may need to Act-As-If more than once. You can use the Act-As-If tool for just about everything in your recovery where you don't feel at ease. This goes for whether you are newly sober or sober awhile.

Recovery and your good life will be easier and will take hold with consistent rituals and habits geared toward sobriety. That's just the way it is. As an addict myself, I want anything that is easier, which means I do rituals and habits which support the recovery and life I want. Even if a ritual is uncomfortable at first, or even a bit boring (to me), it often gets easier and begins to feel good or become relevant over time. If I find, though, any ritual doesn't feel quite right for a period of time, I just find myself another. Recovery Rituals I like that have personal meaning for me make everything easier.

The bigger point about all of this meaning stuff?

Rituals that make no good sense or dampen down your spirit can be exchanged for Recovery Rituals which make sense to you, feel good in your heart, and give your soul permission to come out and play.

Simply put, find the right Recovery Rituals for you.

Find the Experts, Find Your Kind

You may want to find the experts—addicts like you in recovery—who have successfully stayed sober over time and who are living good lives. **Relating to sober addicts like yourself—who have the same addiction—will help you stay sober, feel comforted, and according to one scientific explanation, reduces craving.** As human animals, we need to feel a sense of belonging, like we belong to our herd. When we get around *our* herd, serotonin rises and we feel good because of this rise in our neurochemistry. When addicts are with their kind (alcoholics with alcoholics, gamblers with gamblers, etc.), they feel the herd (a sense of belonging) and with this, good feelings come and craving dissipates.[3] With no craving and with the wonderful feeling that we belong, a sense of safety ensues.

So, what does this all have to do with the importance of rituals and recovery in general? The answer is:

Feeling safe to be ourselves is a large part of recovery.

Think of being a little donkey. You might feel out of place, and maybe a little unsafe, in the middle of a herd of enormous elephants. You, as a donkey, would be even more out of sorts in the middle of a clan of hyenas or a pride of lions. In the midst of these different kinds of animals, you would probably feel terrified. Your terror would trigger an automatic rush of adrenaline. Your brain and body would immediately jolt into gear to kick and run. You would bolt away as fast as you could.

If, though, you put yourself in the middle of a herd of donkeys grazing peacefully in a pasture, you would probably feel good and right. Your body chemistry would relax. There would be no need to run. Your ears could flop a little. Your tail could leisurely swat at flies. You would feel safe and free to be a donkey and would be okay doing what donkeys do.[4]

Once you find your kind of people in recovery, find out what they are doing consistently to stay drug free and satisfied in their life. Then, do what they do. Adopt some of their rituals and practices. They will be your models, and they probably know (from their own experience) that:

Most addicts have a difficult time staying sober all by themselves.

It is much easier to stay sober and happy and in recovery with other recovering addicts who, again, are the true experts. Many of these experts—maybe they aren't donkeys, but human animals like you—are in Twelve Step programs and have successfully stayed sober over time. And lest you think you are joining a cult or some strange organization by being around these people, I guarantee this is not the case. They were all once new to recovery, too—feeling apprehensive, maybe afraid, and possibly a little wary. You may have blocks to being around these odd experts too, and perhaps you have a little judgment. These peculiar people, however, may save your life.

The appeal of the Twelve Step programs is that there are no rules to follow. There are only suggestions you can choose to do or not. You can come and go as you please, believe in a Higher Power or not, and decide how you want to be in recovery. The element of choice is important to recovering addicts (and all people). Choosing rituals within the Twelve Step program design is something reasonable and doable because the element of choice is built in. What anyone does within the Twelve Step program is their own choice.

There are other programs out there though, some church/religious related, some not. The point is, find recovering people (like yourself) that you like and respect, do some of the recovery-related rituals they do, and be consistent. Get with your herd, and when you feel afraid and want to run, get in the middle of your herd. Your herd, even if you like only a few of the donkeys, will help you feel safe.

Rituals Made Easy

Below are some Recovery Rituals. Some are Twelve Step related because of the high success and easily accessible nature of the program. Most are easy to do because you can just show up. You aren't required to do all of them, or any of them. These are just a few examples. How you do your sobriety and what program you choose are your choice. For an easier recovery, though, you will need a few recovery-focused rituals in place with some program that includes contact with other sober people.

Recovery Rituals Could Include

- Weekly attendance at the same recovery meeting (or more than one).
- Talking with a sober buddy regularly.
- Checking in weekly with your sober mentor or sponsor*.
- Going to an outpatient program.
- Talking to someone in your program frequently.
- Working the steps with your sponsor or guide on a consistent basis.
- Introducing yourself to newer people at your meeting.
- Reading program-related or spiritual literature every day.

*A sponsor is a guide of your choosing in the Twelve Step program. This person can help you with the Twelve Steps.

You may notice that all but one of the rituals listed earlier includes being with or making connection with other sober people. There are more than a few reasons why connecting with sober addicts is vital for recovery. Other recovering people light the way of the drug-free path. These people will be of tremendous support.

Also, sober people understand the addict's disconnection from their soul and the world like no one else can. In sobriety, the recovering ones are now part of your fuel for a fun and progressively easier sober existence. The idea that Recovery Rituals include others, as echoed throughout this book, is central to feeling comfortable in one's own recovering skin. **Addicts can't do recovery alone**.

The ritual of reading program-related or spiritual literature every day can't be underestimated as well. This is something done alone or with others. Any program or spiritual reading addresses how to relate to self, others, and something greater than one individual alone. The information—along with quiet reflective time—is also part of what gives rise to an easier recovery. Positive emotions can be jump-started and enhanced by a connection to something greater than oneself. So, alone time too is important.

An easy thing about rituals is that you don't have to reinvent the wheel. Consistent activities are already happening in a recovery community near you. The easy way to do any ritual is to just show up, consistently. That's it. And if you end up somewhere that isn't a good fit for you, choose somewhere else to go. The most important part is finding at least one ritual which involves other sober people—and being consistent with it. Be deliberate. Like the Nike slogan says, "Just do it."

Oh, and one more thing that will make Recovery Rituals and everything else so much easier: Talk to the people at your chosen place, or at least to one person. Remember? We can't do recovery alone. Find someone you like and think you might trust. As you do this, remember that:

Trust is built with someone who has a trustworthy record.

Just because someone is in the program or talks a good talk doesn't mean they are automatically trustworthy. Trust comes with risk, time, and experience. Take time to find and develop a relationship with at least one person who has a trustworthy record with you and with whom you feel safe. Tell this person your secrets. Let this person into the boardroom of your head, where the committee members dwell. This sharing of your innermost self and brain will be crucial for any relief or peace.

Whom Can I Trust?

I remember calling a sober friend once (well, to be rigorously honest, I've called this friend countless times over the years) and talking nonstop for quite a while. In this instance, I was dealing with a relationship problem and was trying, like so many of us do, to figure it out. This friend just listened. No interruptions. It was such a relief to get it all out. She waited until I was completely out of air before saying, "What does Joi want to do?"

Her question stopped me in my tracks. I hadn't thought about what would be good for me in that situation. I knew I could trust her not only because of her own personal track record but also because of her counseling me so wisely over the years. I was lucky. A trustworthy friend and mutual lifelong care were born from the simple Recovery Ritual of calling this person every day in my early sobriety.

When I Trusted the Diet Coach

Speaking of that first year when calling every day seemed a bit much, another incident comes to mind.

I was six months sober, barely 21, and someone was about to stab me in my apartment.

After having grabbed my mustard-colored dial phone with its long extension cord (no cell phones at that time), I slammed my walk-in closet door shut. I was embarrassed to call my sober friend because of a vague thought I might have contributed to the fiasco unfolding around me. And, I thought, *Maybe I deserve to die.* Desperate, though, I decided to call anyway.

Shaking, I told her my story:

I had decided to fast that day because I wanted to lose weight. The diet coach—one of the committee members camped in my head, always weighing in on my food intake—told me I was too fat and insisted I drink only water for 24 hours.

An hour ago, I told my friend, I went to the supermarket for cigarettes and more gallons of water. While there, I thought it would be okay to get a box of those little Entenmann's chocolate chip cookies for later, like tomorrow.

Another committee member in my head—the diet coach's little kid (piping up because the diet coach fell asleep)—convinced me that just one little cookie would be fine, especially since I hadn't eaten all day. I resisted for about a second and then decided to open the box of bite-sized little buggers while in the store and have just one, maybe two.

Before I knew it, I had wolfed down the entire box and woke up at the refrigerator case looking for cottage cheese to balance out my blood sugar. Apparently, the diet coach had woken up during my sugar-induced blackout and insisted protein would fix the situation. At this point (I admitted to my friend, still listening on the line), I was feeling a bit panicky but believed cottage cheese would calm me down. The diet coach told me so.

Then, on my way to purchase my Marlboros and water, I stuffed the empty cookie box behind a shelf, making sure no one was peering around the aisle, although I thought this might be a possibility. People always seemed to be lurking about in the aisles. Coast clear, I scurried to the checkout counter, paid for the cigarettes, water, and cottage cheese—but not for the cookies in my belly. I hustled out of there quick.

On my drive home, stuffing my face with the cottage cheese with a grungy plastic spoon I was grateful to have found in the glove compartment, I kept my eyes fixed to the rearview mirror. I knew a car was following me. My breath quickened.

I figured the aisle-peering people saw I had left the store without paying for the cookies, and now one was going to bust into my apartment and kill me, like in some horror movie. I swore I heard someone breathing right outside my closet door. The mustard phone cord felt like someone was yanking on it. I was hyperventilating at this point when my friend told me to breathe.

My friend talked me through this (what felt like a psychotic) episode. As it turned out, no one was following me, and no one was out to kill me.

All of the members that contributed to the little drama—the diet coach, little kid, cookie thief, and paranoid one—all had a big say in my life that night and taught me a big lesson:

When the committee starts up, I can do what they say and be a little (or a lot) crazy, or I can be the boss of me (and them) and be sane. As my friend said that night, **"You can do anything you want as long as you are willing to pay the price."**

I didn't exactly know what Joi wanted to do for a long time, but one thing she didn't want was a redo of that night. I went on a lot of suspicious diets after that but never fasted again.

How great it is to have a trusted other with whom we can sort out our relationships, diet dramas, and everything else. Without accessing such help, there is a good chance the most insufferable, compulsive, or frightened committee member may take over and hold you hostage in your own closet.

By having some good Recovery Rituals and talking to at least one person with whom you can share a bit about your addiction and challenges, you will have already arrived at the next cornerstone in the cycle: Contrary Action.

Recovery Recap

- Recovery Rituals are consistent activities that support a recovery program meaningful to you.
- Recovery Rituals promote abstinence, structure, and good feelings.
- Recovery Rituals are often easily accessible and will connect you to sober people like yourself.
- You get to choose rituals with personal meaning that you like.
- You may want to Act-As-If for a while when settling on a Recovery Ritual—it is okay and normal to feel a little (or a lot) uncomfortable when beginning any new experience.
- Find your sober herd and do what they do—these are the experts who can help you feel safe and free to be YOU.
- Addicts cannot do recovery alone.
- Doing a Recovery Ritual is easy—just show up.
- Trust is built over time with someone who has a trustworthy record.
- It is crucial to find at least one trustworthy, sober person in whom you can confide.

Clinician's Corner

A discussion about recovery tools and resources in a clinical setting is helpful for recovering people, especially when clients report trauma and family dysfunction. From what I've seen, though, we see more abstinence and a higher quality of emotional sobriety when therapy is combined with Recovery Rituals outside the 50-minute hour.

The addict brain may try to talk the addict feet out of doing any Recovery Ritual. Ideally, the recovering person will learn how to have smart feet instead of relying solely on their brain (and/or yours) when it comes to accessing help.

If you sense any resistance in adopting Recovery Rituals, back up and assess your client for willingness, using David Burns' Willingness Scale.[5] This therapist's tool is a winner and I highly suggest you check it out.

As usual, you answer the following questions too, modifying for the thing you gave up for the duration of reading this book.

Step Into Your Life (15–20 Minutes Plus Field Time)

Write out your answers.

1. Name two Recovery Rituals you will commit to do, one which includes other people, the other an alone time practice. What are your feelings about, or reasons for, these rituals? How do they speak to you personally?
2. Have you ever Acted-As-If? Describe. If not, do you think you will try this? For what?
3. What are your thoughts about the idea that recovering people can't recover alone?
4. Do you have one trustworthy person with whom you can confide? How do you know you can trust this person?

Field time: Choose a Recovery Ritual, do it, and report back to your trustworthy person, if you have one.

Straight Shot (3–5 Minutes)

1. Name one Recovery Ritual you will commit to do.
2. What is the value of this Recovery Ritual for you? What purpose does it serve? Why is it important to you?

Notes

1. "It Works, But Why Does It Work? Perspectives on Change in 12-Step and Non-12-Step Mutual-Help Groups," Recovery Research Institute, accessed December 20, 2021, www.recoveryanswers.org/research-post/why-does-it-work-perspectives-change-12-step-non-12-step-mutual-help-groups/. Evidence suggests that greater involvement with mutual-help groups (a.k.a. self-help/peer support groups typically run by volunteers where recovery experiences and skills are shared) have better recovery outcomes.
2. A "life script" is a life plan developed subconsciously in childhood that governs how we live our lives. The term was defined by Eric Berne, creator of transactional analysis, a popular psychological theory in the 1960s and 70s. Before recovery, life scripts are often filled with some extreme form of tragedy, melodrama, or the like, brought on by the addict's decisions. These decisions are in response to negative beliefs taken on (subconsciously) in childhood. In recovery, beliefs about ourselves, others, and the world can be transformed from adverse to affirming—we can do rewrites if we want to change the tone of our lives. It is in the rewriting that we learn to do good and feel good.
3. Ronald A. Ruden and Marcia Byalick, *The Craving Brain*, 2nd ed. (New York: Harper, 2003), 94–96.
4. fredjoiners, "The AA Camel Story," *Alcoholics Anonymous Cleveland*, accessed December 20, 2021, www.aacle.org/the-aa-camel-story/. For any recovery history enthusiasts out there, the camel, also a herd animal, is considered the sobriety symbol for Alcoholics Anonymous. Dr. Bob, cofounder of Alcoholics Anonymous with Bill Wilson, would refer to the camel when discussing prayer.
5. David Burns, *Feeling Great: The Revolutionary New Treatment for Depression and Anxiety* (Eau Claire, WI: PESI Publishing & Media, 2020), 21. Burns, author of many books, has created numerous assessment scales. His Willingness Test, although designed for depression and anxiety, may give you some idea of your client's willingness around Recovery Rituals. To access the Willingness Test, see page 21 here: www.readpbn.com/pdf/Feeling-Great-The-Revolutionary-New-Treatment-for-Depression-and-Anxiety-Sample-Pages.pdf. Swap out the word "exercises" for Recovery Rituals and see how your client answers.

Works Cited

Burns, David. *Feeling Great: The Revolutionary New Treatment for Depression and Anxiety*. Eau Claire, WI: PESI Publishing & Media, 2020.

fredjoiners. "The AA Camel Story." *Alcoholics Anonymous Cleveland*. Accessed December 20, 2021. www.aacle.org/the-aa-camel-story/.

Recovery Research Institute. "It Works, But Why Does It Work? Perspectives on Change in 12-Step and Non-12-Step Mutual-Help Groups." Accessed December 20, 2021. www.recoveryanswers.org/research-post/why-does-it-work-perspectives-change-12-step-non-12-step-mutual-help-groups/.

Ruden, Ronald A., and Marcia Byalick. *The Craving Brain*. 2nd ed. New York: HarperCollins, 2000.

5 If Nothing Changes, Nothing Changes

In This Chapter

- What is Contrary Action?
- Vignettes: An Alcoholic, Overeater/Debtor, and Sex Addict Take Contrary Action
- Out of Your Comfort Zone and Into Your Life

Contrary Action, the third cornerstone in the Recovery Cycle, opens the door to so much in life. With taking some emotional risks, healing and love become more available. With Contrary Action, recovering people can look forward to repairing existing relationships and building new ones, along with so much more.

What Is Contrary Action?

Contrary Action—at its most basic—**is making a conscious choice to do something other than habitual self-destructive behavior**. This means doing something different than you would normally do. Also, **Contrary Action is positive action** even though it might not feel normal or comfortable.

Abstinence is the first and most important Contrary Action for the addict. Can you think of the reason this might be?

The answer is: Recovery begins with abstinence.

Remember: The normal state for an addict is to be using. Abstinence is contrary—or opposite—of what the addict would normally do. To take the Contrary Action of being abstinent produces different results—positive results—in the sober person's life. In the beginning days of sobriety, it becomes apparent that:

With abstinence, there can be recovery and a good life.

We see others in recovery are living these good lives, especially if we have a few good Recovery Rituals in place. These others are not just talking about abstinence, though.

DOI: 10.4324/9781003293231-8

The concept of Contrary Action doesn't just apply to abstinence.[1] Abstinence plus doing some things differently in your life will be necessary if you want recovery that is meaningful, joyful, and full of growth. That said, Contrary Action will apply to many situations over the course of a recovery plan. The overarching idea of Contrary Action is that recovery requires we stretch in new ways.

Vignettes: An Alcoholic, Overeater/Debtor, and Sex Addict Take Contrary Action

See how Randy, Maria, and Steve's Contrary Action helped them ultimately feel better about themselves and grow in self-esteem.

Randy (Alcoholic) Walks Through Fear

Randy is in his early 30s and three months sober off alcohol and marijuana. He has been attending AA meetings the entire time he has been sober. Ever since Randy can remember, he has been afraid of people and what they think of him. He sits in the back row at the meetings, laughs at some of the shares, and has heard people talking about their sponsors. He wants a sponsor but has been afraid to ask anyone. He's heard some stories about how people get a sponsor and has hoped someone will magically appear and ask him if he wants a sponsor. His normal way is to wait for people to come talk to him because he is so afraid and anxious. His last girlfriend called him "habitually passive."

At a meeting one day, a man sitting next to Randy asks him if he has a sponsor. Randy replies, "Not yet." The person then asks, "Do you want a sponsor?"

Randy, feeling a bit cornered but hopeful says, "Yes." The truth, though, is part of him wants a sponsor but another part of him doesn't.

The man says, "I think Liam would make a good sponsor for you. Why don't you go and ask him now?"

Randy, feeling deflated thinks, *Why doesn't this guy just mind his own business and leave me alone?*

The man nudges him and says, "Go on, do it."

Randy gets up and walks up to Liam. Terrified, he mumbles, "Hi, Liam, um . . . would you consider sponsoring me?"

Much to Randy's surprise, Liam says, "Sure!" Randy is amazed at how relieved he feels.

Months after asking Liam to be his sponsor, Randy can't believe how good and supported he feels. Now, he walks up to newer people at meetings and introduces himself. He now experiences this as easy and feels good about himself doing it.

The Contrary Action Randy took—walking up to Liam in spite of how afraid he was—bore fruit. He felt relieved and supported. Normally Randy would hide in his own life by drinking and smoking dope. Now sober and working with a sponsor, he is taking risks and doing things differently—positive things—which are resulting in more good feelings and positive results.

Maria (Overeater and Debtor) Learns to Have Fun

Maria, in her mid-40s, is sober off sugar and in Overeaters Anonymous for five years and has been in Debtors Anonymous for two years. Maria is a successful executive and works most weekends. She has always wanted to ride her bike as a hobby but tells herself she doesn't have time.

One day, Maria was complaining to a friend in recovery that she was going to work all weekend but would love to go biking instead. The friend said, "You work every weekend. Don't you ever plan time for fun and something you like to do?"

Maria replied, "I go to the movies on Saturday nights, or catch up on work."

"Yeah, but you say you want to go biking. When are you going to do that, when you're in heaven?"

Both laughed but Maria got the point. Her overworking had been pointed out to her before. But this time she heard it and decided to take Contrary Action and do her weekend time differently. She planned a bike ride in the hills near her house for a few hours on the next Saturday.

During the ride, she totally forgot about work and had a great time enjoying the sunshine and exercise. She wondered why she hadn't been taking this special time for herself all along.

Later, Maria realized her work didn't suffer. In fact, she seemed to get more done and had more energy. She liked it so much she made a plan to make it a weekly thing, and even began thinking about taking a biking vacation.

Maria came to discover that the Contrary Action of scheduling something fun for herself was good for her spirit. She experienced the positive results of doing something she normally would deny herself. With this new action of biking on the weekend, she felt energized and more relaxed at the same time. This was certainly a positive thing in her sobriety.

Steve (Sex Addict) Gets Honest and Experiences Feeling Honorable

Steve, a recovering sex addict in his late 40s, has a daughter who hasn't spoken to him in two years because of his transgressions outside of the home. He has not acted out for one year and wants to find a way to re-establish the relationship with his daughter. He feels ashamed and guilty and is terrified the daughter won't accept him back into her life. He is also afraid the mother, his ex-wife, will contaminate his attempt. A deeper fear is that he isn't cut out to be a good father and he judges himself a horrible man and not worthy of a relationship with his daughter. *How could I face her?* he thinks.

Steve, up until this time, had shared only bits and pieces of his story with his Sexaholics Anonymous sponsor. One day though, deep, painful feelings started to rumble and surface. With this issue, Steve felt an agonizing pain in his heart—he had to tell someone or he would go back to his compulsive behavior. Steve didn't want to go back to acting out, though, so he decided to take a risk and share the pain, shame, and details of his sexual history with his sponsor. It was the first time he had discussed his entire story with anyone, including how he felt about his mother, his daughter, and all women, and his thinking that no one—especially women—could ever love and accept him. He let it all out, and this was cathartic and weirdly freeing.

Rather than keeping the pain to himself, Steve took Contrary Action, sought help from his sponsor, and felt better. Feeling better was a positive result. But he knew there would be more Contrary Action needed for recovery to take hold.

The sponsor told Steve making amends was certainly due to his daughter and ex-wife, but before that, there was other work to do. The sponsor asked Steve to do an inventory and to include all of his fears in this inventory.[2] The sponsor laid out the rest of the process that would happen before Steve would get the green light to make his amends.[3] The sponsor also suggested Steve get some therapy for the underlying roots of his sex addiction. With all of this Steve felt queasy yet hopeful.

Steve continued the work suggested by the sponsor, and the sponsor acknowledged that Steve was growing into an honorable man. This helped Steve *feel* honorable. He knew in his gut he was laying a solid foundation for his sober future. The thought to act out sexually became more and more distant. In a way, he was desensitizing to both the painful feelings from his past and the good feelings around being a sober man who was now honest and doing the right thing. This was sometimes uncomfortable but easier than going back to his addiction and isolation.

Steve thought everything he was doing was Contrary Action because it all was uncomfortable at first. Whereas before he led a secretive existence, now he was telling the truth about his pain, shame, and fears to another man who understood and didn't judge him. Soon enough, though, Steve began to experience that with sound guidance, working through his problems was much easier than holding it all in alone. Everything became easier with his sponsor, the support of the men in the program, and his therapist's guidance. Steve continued to make positive choices in his recovery and today is beginning to communicate with his daughter.

Out of Your Comfort Zone and Into Your Life

Contrary Action might be outside your comfort zone because you may not be used to doing things in a more positive, rational way, especially if you are newer in recovery. Even if you have some sober time under your belt, doing something more positive may be uncomfortable for you too.

Addicts tend toward self-destruction, even if the self-destruction doesn't come in the form of using. Again, normal for the addict is to be drunk and then feel bad about it. Making decisions that are self-destructive, where the payoff is pain, is almost habitual. We get high from the pain. This could be part of the reason people in recovery do some crazy things where they end up feeling bad about themselves.

It's as if we've found a way to use without using! We seem to find a way to squash joy, as if we aren't worthy or don't deserve a joyful life. This often has to do with faulty belief systems (i.e., negative thinking patterns about self, others, and reality). Putting a microscope on one's negative thoughts and evaluating them can be helpful, and part of what the "cognitive" in cognitive behavioral therapy is all about. But we could get stuck thinking "isn't it awful," maybe in a therapist's office, looking at how bad our thoughts make us feel. Or, we can look at those same thoughts and then get to work on changing something.

This is where the Contrary Action part of the cycle comes in to save the day and save your life in recovery. Any discomfort you may feel in doing Contrary Action will likely morph into more self-esteem, relief, fun, and joy. This is part of healing in recovery. The behavioral part. **We must stretch and change our self-destructive behaviors to self-affirming ones if we want to grow in self-esteem and enjoy life in recovery**. With this stretching, we learn we can feel good and expand our ability to do so.

In life, we will experience painful feelings. No doubt about that. Expect some pain. Keep in mind, though, that the ultimate payoff of doing Contrary Action even if painful or uncomfortable will ultimately result in you feeling good about you, and that good feelings will return. And everything is easier when we feel good, right?

Practical Examples of Contrary Action

There are an infinite number of examples for Contrary Action, depending on individual circumstances. Table 5.1 shows a few examples. Some examples are about avoiding the addiction, while others are about other life challenges.

Individual circumstances will dictate what Contrary Action is needed. Everyone's recovery is a little different. Honor your own temperament, history, and life situation.

You can choose to be the same you, or you can choose to stretch in a new way. If you don't like where you are in your recovery and you want something to change, then take some Contrary Action to change it. Remember, "If nothing changes, nothing changes."

Table 5.1 Practical examples of Contrary Action.

Old Behavior	Contrary Action
Driving by the dealer's house or usual liquor store on your way home	Driving a different way home to avoid being triggered
Calling a friend with whom you used to get high	Making a call to a sober friend
Binging on ice cream after dinner	Going for a walk after dinner
Isolating as you ruminate about a problem	Calling a friend to do something fun, or calling your sponsor to get some feedback about your problem
Getting to your recovery meeting late	Getting to your recovery meeting early to help set up and talk to others
Giving the finger to someone on the freeway who cuts you off	Continuing to drive normally, keeping your hands on the wheel and remembering to breathe
Not going back to school because you think you are too old or not smart enough	Signing up for one class at the community college
Never asking a girl on a date because you are afraid she'll say no	Asking a girl on a date
Flipping from one relationship to another every month	Not dating for a year
Telling your boss he's a jerk	Calling a sober person to vent and talk it out when you are angry about your boss or job
Putting your fist through the drywall when angry	Leaving the room to cool off/take a time out before responding

In the next chapter we will explore Connection which, if you look back at the Recovery Cycle, is the delicious fruit underneath Contrary Action. If you want to learn more about this nourishing recovery sugar, keep reading. **Yes, there is a healthy sugar—the sweet relationships we get to have in recovery**.

Recovery Recap

- Contrary Action is taking positive action (rather than self-destructive action).
- The most important Contrary Action in recovery is abstinence.
- After abstinence there are an infinite number of Contrary Actions one can take, depending on individual circumstances.
- Taking Contrary Action is not always comfortable.
- By taking Contrary Action, we stretch so we can grow into the life we want and experience healing from addiction.
- We expand our ability to feel good and grow in self-esteem by taking Contrary Action, even if it seems uncomfortable or painful in some way at the time.
- "If nothing changes, nothing changes."

Clinician's Corner

Assisting addicts to take Contrary Action can be challenging! Limiting beliefs can be fervent, cunning, and conquering in nature and can inhibit clients from living the life they want. One theory suggests we have either a growth mindset or a fixed mindset.[4] Simply put, a person with a fixed mindset avoids new challenges and learning, whereas a person with a growth mindset embraces them, considering the bigger picture. Let your clients know that by participating in new affirming activities (i.e., taking Contrary Action), they will change the neural pathways in their brains and begin to inhabit the good life they want.[5] Remind them that discomfort might be expected with some Contrary Action, but eventually good feelings, self-esteem, and confidence grow.

As usual, you do the exercise, too.

Novel (Neural) Paths (15–20 Minutes Plus Field Time)

Write out your answers.

1. Now that you've taken the Contrary Action of abstinence, what positive outcomes have you experienced? List.
2. What other Contrary Actions have you taken in your recovery? What happened?
3. Describe a significant Contrary Action that would be a step in a direction you want to go (instead of doing what you normally do). In what ways would this Contrary Action be good for you?
4. For the Contrary Action you listed earlier, who would you choose to support you so you could bookend your experience? (Meaning, you would discuss your experience with them before and after taking the Contrary Action.) Now, tell that person about what you want to do.
5. Field time: Do what you identified in #4, and report back to that person.

Straight Shot (5 Minutes Plus Field Time)

1. Choose a Contrary Action you are willing to take and discuss it with your therapist, sober support person or group.
2. Do it, and report back to your support.

Notes

1. Rebecca E. Williams and Julie S. Kraft, *The Mindfulness Workbook for Addiction: A Guide to Coping with the Grief, Stress and Anger that Trigger Addictive Behaviors* (Oakland, CA: New Harbinger, 2012), 51–57. Williams and Craft have an exercise in their workbook called "Choosing the Opposite," borrowing a skill from a concept based on a *dialectical behavior therapy* (DBT), created by Marsha Linehan. This

workbook is a wonderful tool for developing healthy coping skills while avoiding emotional triggers.

2. *Alcoholics Anonymous*, 4th ed. (New York: Alcoholics Anonymous World Services, 2001), 59. An inventory is referred to in the Twelve Step programs as the Fourth Step (i.e., "Made a searching and fearless moral inventory of ourselves"). This is where the recovering person reflects on their part in reaction to people, places, and things and puts this in writing. The idea is to examine resentments along with one's part in relationships, circumstances, behaviors, and thinking. Simply put, an inventory is about taking an honest look at the not-so-good and good parts of oneself in great detail, along with listing one's fears.

3. Ibid. Step Nine in the Twelve Step programs is "Made direct amends to such people wherever possible, except when to do so would injure them or others." The intent of Step Nine is that the recovering person cleans up their own side of the street and amends any past behavior that caused another (or oneself) harm. Before making any amends, the addict is advised to work the preceding steps with a sponsor or guide and get counsel on how to make amends.

4. Carol S. Dweck, *Mindset: The New Psychology of Success—How We Can Learn to Fulfill Our Full Potential* (New York: Random House, 2016).

5. Eagle Gamma, "What is Brain Plasticity? Also Known as Neuroplasticity," *Simply-Psychology*, March 23, 2021, www.simplypsychology.org/brain-plasticity.html.

Works Cited

Alcoholics Anonymous. *Alcoholics Anonymous: Big Book Reference Edition for Addiction Treatment*. 4th ed. New York: Alcoholics Anonymous, 2014.

Dweck, Carol S. *Mindset: The New Psychology of Success—How We Can Learn to Fulfill Our Full Potential*. New York: Random House, 2016.

Eagle Gamma. "What Is Brain Plasticity? Also Known as Neuroplasticity." *SimplyPsychology*. March 23, 2021. www.simplypsychology.org/brain-plasticity.html.

Williams, Rebecca E., and Julie S. Kraft. *The Mindfulness Workbook for Addiction: A Guide to Coping With the Grief, Stress and Anger that Trigger Addictive Behaviors*. Oakland, CA: New Harbinger, 2012.

6 Comfort in Recovery

In This Chapter

- What Is Connection?
- Why Is Connection Important?
- Your Golden Ticket to Good Feelings
- Connected in Love

The sound bite, "The opposite of addiction is connection,"[1] struck a chord for many and reverberated into a statement that addiction is not a substance abuse disorder but a social disorder.[2] Positive social connection is certainly a huge part of recovery—even for devout introverts—but the opposite of addiction is more nuanced than these two ideas suggest.[3]

As echoed throughout this book, addicts will need to *do* something to move away from addiction/isolation and toward recovery/connection. Societal and communal mechanisms will help in prevention, for sure, but until that perfect social order is in place, the recovering person will want to plug themselves into recovery with others as they discover the "why" of their addiction and the "how" of doing life sober. This book, as said earlier, is mostly about the how.[4]

A true connection with others and the world in a positive way is possible—and doable—no matter what the social circumstance, genetic disposition, psychological challenge, or spiritual view.

As you read through this chapter, think about how connection relates to recovery.

What Is Connection?

Connection—in a basic sense—means related or linked.

Connection—in a more specific recovery sense—**means the recovering person feels related to others and the world in a good way because he is now in honest relationship with self, others, and something greater than oneself.**

Note: This "something greater than oneself" is referred to as a Higher Power in the Twelve Step programs but could be anything greater than you with more power than your own brain, no matter what program you choose. Some

DOI: 10.4324/9781003293231-9

recovering people have no problem with the idea of a Higher Power, while others might bristle and quail, thinking the Twelve Step program religious, or that a Higher Power is a punishing God (or something of the sort). This is not the case. A Higher Power is all about how you understand it. You can call it whatever you want. Maybe your word would be Mother Nature or Spirit. More on all of this in Chapter 10, though.

With Connection, the recovering person is not cut off from self or others. (Like our donkey friend from earlier, he has found his herd.) He is not alone with his thoughts, feelings, and whatever else is rattling around in his active brain. He is in relationship with others. He chooses these relationships, and these connections are positive. He connects to guidance, support, and sober friendships. When with others, or even with just one other sober person that gets him, he feels good and safe. He appreciates the positive connections and comes to rely on the good feelings, understanding, and support these special people provide.

Why Is Connection Important?

Have you ever had an experience that everything was okay in that moment? Maybe the feeling was joy, or serenity, or happiness. Or maybe it was feeling satisfied or comforted in some way, or that you were just, well, *connected*. Did this feeling of Connection just happen? Were you using? Were you sober?

Connection must be experienced to appreciate its importance. I can do my best to give you reasons why I think this Connection and relatedness are vital to a thriving recovery, but until you experience this for yourself, it will just be a theory or words. I will do my best to answer the question from my own experience.

A False Sense of Connection

I experienced what I thought was a true connected feeling with my first drink. At the time, pursuing this connection through alcohol and cocaine seemed harmless. When I was under the influence, people understood me, or so I thought. I felt normal. I could talk to people. As I ferociously played Yahtzee all night long with other addicts, all worries, insecurities, and fears slipped away (until I heard the birds chirping in the morning, after which I needed a Valium to take the stark reality, paranoia, and demoralization away).

This connection, however skewed and fleeting, was a feeling that allowed me to feel free and open to the world and others—as long as I had enough cocaine and alcohol to last forever. The problem was, there was never enough. I kept chasing that connected feeling with whatever drugs were available, but that special feeling faded away the more I pursued it. Long after it had disappeared, I wondered why I was still chasing it in my closet all alone under a pile of dirty laundry and empty beer cans.

Obviously, that connection wasn't real. The people didn't really understand me at all. No one had a clue that I desperately needed to feel connected and what I really wanted was to feel connected and okay—without using.

At that time, I often wondered if people really lived their lives feeling connected and comfortable. Were people just faking it and not admitting they felt weirdly disconnected like me? Or worse, was everyone comfortable and I was freakishly alone?

Real Connection

When I quit drinking and using, I began to feel a sense of real Connection just by hanging around sober people and talking and laughing with them. The laughter helped a lot. Most were nothing like me in any way. These recovering addicts weren't using, though, and strangely, because we shared the addiction problem and a common solution to our problem, I could relate to them. I had a felt sense that they could relate to me as well.

In the sharing of stories with these like-minded people and together finding solutions to our problems, I felt connected to people in a good way. To keep this Connection though, I needed to stay abstinent, continue to engage in rituals I liked, AND do more Contrary Action.

Contrary Action in the beginning was talking to other sober people. I did this, even though it felt uncomfortable. Little by little I started feeling some of those good feelings—comfort especially—and that everything was going to be okay. With more and more Contrary Action in other areas of my life, I began to feel connected in an even deeper way.

As this deeper Connection evolved, the realization came that it was spiritual in nature. Getting to know oneself, having a deepening Connection with a Force greater than me, and a growing acceptance of oneself and others, is part of this Connection. Being increasingly comfortable with where we fit in life and in our communities is another outgrowth of this Connection. This Connection helps us feel safe, that everything is okay, and that everything is going to be okay, and that yes, we are all connected in some profound way. This shared Spirit is our safety net. It is available to us at all times and is a large part of what constitutes a feeling of awe and overall well-being in recovery, even when having a bad patch of feelings. All of this without a psychedelic drug.

Have you ever felt connected in a similar way? Or, if you've had your own feeling of Connection can you describe it? Do you have reasons why this Connection is important for you?

Your Golden Ticket to Good Feelings

Remember the Addiction Cycle? If you look at it again (in Chapter 1 or in the Appendix), you will see Isolation just underneath Using. Do you remember how you felt during one of your last awful binges? Did you feel alone with your demoralization? Or just plain alone and isolated but not in a good way?

Isolation, a direct consequence of Using, only results in not feeling good. Once you've experienced this Isolation and know deep down you have a problem with addiction, there is no going back to being a normal drinker, a moderate gambler, a person not addicted to porn, or whatever kind of addict you are. You have the allergy-like ailment. If you use, you will eventually end up isolated and feeling bad in some way, and/or a significant relationship will suffer. If you are interested in living drug free, though, Connection is available and will make your recovery so much easier than going it alone. Good feelings come with Connection and:

> **The golden ticket to your good feelings will be in the supportive relationships you make and Contrary Action you take.**

Taking a risk on reaching out to someone for help is a vital Contrary Action. This is how we build positive, sober, human connection and learn to feel good.

Connected in Love

As said earlier, establishing supportive relationships in recovery comes from doing some Contrary Action, even if it doesn't feel comfortable at the time. When we find we feel accepted in these relationships, this acceptance fosters a sense of love in us. We begin to feel loved and learn how to love others. No more are we isolated alone. We become connected in love and more lovable.

A Love Connection

Working through new, strange, and mixed feelings is part of sobriety just as it is for anyone, addict or not. With consistent practice, allowing others to support us feels good. This support—this Connection—helps us feel and accept the new universe of feelings we are bound to experience in recovery. Experiencing feelings is part of being human. And in recovery, we get to feel love and share love in relatedness. A growing love of self and others is central to recovery and our day-to-day living.

> **Connection helps us in becoming feeling, functioning people who can experience love in relationship.**

Do you know anyone who doesn't want to feel more love in their life? And what about you, do you want the experience of feeling and sharing love?

Will Connection Help Me Feel Better?

If you are still wondering if Connection is something you want, and you are unsure if it will help you feel better, maybe the following questions will help you:

- Do you want to feel more love in your life?
- Have you ever wanted an aching loneliness to go away?
- When you are having a rough time, do you want to feel better?
- Do you feel a spiritual void?
- Do you wish you had a friend that understood?
- Is there a secret you want to get out?
- Have you thought something is holding you back from being yourself or accomplishing something?
- Are you afraid of people?
- Do you regret the past?
- Do you want to know how to have a loving relationship?

If you answered "Yes" to at least two of these questions, Connection will most likely help you feel better.

If my idea of Connection (or your sense of what it might feel like) appeals to you, then the most important question is: Are you willing to take an emotional risk (by taking Contrary Action) to get it? If yes, ask someone for help. For sure it might be risky and uncomfortable to take Contrary Action. No doubt about that. But doing something different—not your usual way—may be better than going it alone. Addicts really do need support. All of us. This support helps us feel more comfortable in recovery.

If you are having difficulty getting this concept of Connection and the spiritual nature of it, maybe ask someone in your program or another sober friend what Connection means to them, and how they got it. Ask if they feel comforted and supported. Tell this person what you do or don't understand about what you've read or experienced. Maybe this would be Contrary Action for you. Perhaps some feelings would come up. You might have some uncomfortable feelings, or maybe some good feelings, or possibly a little of both. That's okay. Feelings are what the next chapter is all about, so if you read on, you will be prepared for any feeling you might have should you decide to stretch and risk doing something out of your comfort zone.

Recovery Recap

- Connection means being linked to others and the world in a way that feels good and positive—it is the opposite of feeling achingly isolated.
- Connection comes with being in honest relationship with self, others, and something greater than oneself.
- The golden ticket to your good feelings will be in the supportive relationships you make and Contrary Action you take.

- Your feeling of Connection is experiential, to be discovered, felt, and defined by you.
- Connection helps us become feeling, functioning people who can experience love in relationships.
- Connection will help you feel better.
- Connection will only come with taking some emotional risks that will (most likely) be Contrary Action for you.

Clinician's Corner

To walk in your client's shoes, you must imagine the terror many addicted people feel around the idea of connecting with other recovering people. Isolation has practically been a way of life, so engaging with others in an honest, meaningful way may trigger great fear.

This fear can appear masked in resistance, rebelliousness, denial, gallows laughter, or excessive niceness. If you create a safe place for your clients, you have an opportunity to assist them in raising their consciousness around fears that keep them stuck. In other words, if they feel safe enough to be honest, they may feel more connected to themselves, and therefore more willing to connect with other sober peers for support. You cannot be your client's sole recovery support.

Also, it's good to remember evidence-based research that concludes, "A number of relationship factors—such as agreeing on therapy goals, getting client feedback throughout the course of treatment, and repairing ruptures—are at least as vital to a positive outcome as using the right treatment method."[5] Basically, find a way to connect with your partner—with this, your client may be more inclined to do the recovery work.

Now, think about how you've felt abstaining from the thing you decided to give up at the beginning of this book and answer the subsequent questions, as usual, before giving them to your clients. If you don't attend a program, consider sharing your answers with your supervision group, a peer clinician, a supervisor, or a therapist.

Moving Toward Connection (20–30 Minutes)

Answer the questions in writing or have your client answer in session.

1. What is your experience with feeling Connection in recovery? Do you feel connected or disconnected? To whom? Explain.

2. Do you feel afraid to connect to a program or anyone in it? If yes, what are you afraid of? Is there someone you want to reach out to? If yes, what has prevented you from doing so? If you have connected to a program or a sober person, describe your experience.

3. Pick one of the questions under the *Will Connection Help Me Feel Better* section, where you answered yes. What are your reasons for the yes? Are you willing to share this with someone?

4. What are your thoughts about the quote, "The opposite of addiction is connection?"

5. Share your answers with your therapist or sober guide.

Straight Shot (3–5 Minutes)

1. Go up to someone you want to connect with at a recovery meeting and ask them how they are. Stay with that person for at least 3 minutes or more. Or tell your therapist your greatest fear about connecting with someone in a recovery group.

Notes

1. Johann Hari, "Everything You Think You Know About Addiction Is Wrong," *TED Talk Video*, June 2015, www.ted.com/talks/johann_hari_everything_you_think_you_know_about_addiction_is_wrong.

2. Robert Weiss, "The Opposite of Addiction Is Connection," *Psychology Today*, September 30, 2015, www.psychologytoday.com/us/blog/love-and-sex-in-the-digital-age/201509/the-opposite-addiction-is-connection.

3. Amanda L. Giordano, "What Exactly Is the Biopsychosocial Model of Addiction?" (para. 1), *Psychology Today*, July 10, 2021, www.psychologytoday.com/ca/blog/understanding-addiction/202107/what-exactly-is-the-biopsychosocial-model-addiction. "The biopsychosocial model of addiction provides a holistic, multifaceted conceptualization of the disorder. Rather than one cause, numerous biological, psychological, and social factors increase or decrease the risk of addiction among

individuals. Genetics, biology, mental health concerns, trauma, social norms, and availability all contribute to the risk of addiction."

4. Annie Hunt, "Expanding the Biopsychosocial Model: The Active Reinforcement Model of Addiction," *Graduate Student Journal of Psychology* 15 (2014): 57–69, www.tc.columbia.edu/publications/gsjp/gsjp-volumes-archive/36306_5Hunt.pdf. Whereas the biopsychosocial model of addiction addresses underlying causes of addiction, the active reinforcement model of addiction posits that addiction is sustained by (a) impaired neurological mechanisms, (b) unmet psychological needs, and (c) dysfunctional behavior, and that these elements are interdependent. The idea here? This more comprehensive model may generate more successful treatment outcomes because clinicians can address (and maybe even predict) how one element affects another. In other words, clinicians can (a) carefully unravel the threads of addiction without forcing the pull on one thread, and (b) help clients sew their new recovery robes in a sober fashion that works for them.

5. Tori DeAngelis, "Better Relationships with Patients Lead to Better Outcomes," *Monitor on Psychology* 50, no. 10 (2019): 38, www.apa.org/monitor/2019/11/ce-corner-relationships. Article about the APA Task Force on Evidence-Based Relationships and Responsiveness study of 16 meta-analyses on aspects of the therapy relationship.

Works Cited

DeAngelis, Tori. "Better Relationships with Patients Lead to Better Outcomes." *Monitor on Psychology* 50, no. 10 (2019): 38. www.apa.org/monitor/2019/11/ce-corner-relationships.

Giordano, Amanda L. "What Exactly Is the Biopsychosocial Model of Addiction?" *Psychology Today.* July 10, 2021. www.psychologytoday.com/ca/blog/understanding-addiction/202107/what-exactly-is-the-biopsychosocial-model-addiction.

Hari, Johann. "Everything You Think You Know About Addiction Is Wrong." *TED Talk Video.* June 2015. www.ted.com/talks/johann_hari_everything_you_think_you_know_about_addiction_is_wrong.

Hunt, Annie. "Expanding the Biopsychosocial Model: The Active Reinforcement Model of Addiction." *Graduate Student Journal of Psychology* 15 (2014): 57–69. www.tc.columbia.edu/publications/gsjp/gsjp-volumes-archive/36306_5Hunt.pdf.

Weiss, Robert. "The Opposite of Addiction is Connection." *Psychology Today.* September 30, 2015. www.psychologytoday.com/us/blog/love-and-sex-in-the-digital-age/201509/the-opposite-addiction-is-connection.

7 Feeling Feelings, Being Human

In This Chapter

- What Is a Range of Feelings?
- Are Feelings Important?
- Impulse Control and Naming Feelings
- Desensitizing to Feelings
- Too Much Emphasis on Feelings?
- Choosing Guides

This chapter presents how to acknowledge, name, and accept an expanded Range of Feelings. With this, recovering people (and all people, really) are in a better position to make a positive decision about what they want (or don't want) to do. To live in the Recovery Cycle, addicts move on after giving their feelings attention, honor, and credibility.

What Is a Range of Feelings?

A Range of Feelings, which is the fourth cornerstone of the Recovery Cycle, **means you will experience many different feelings the longer you are in recovery.** This is good news and sometimes not-so-good news for sober people. The good news? The aching demoralization and loneliness are replaced with the satisfaction of staying sober and feeling connected in a good way. The not-so-good news? All kinds of feelings—even the uncomfortable and deeply painful ones—are part of a drug-free life too. This is normal and to be expected.

We all like good feelings but painful feelings hurt. Still, just because something feels painful doesn't necessarily mean pain is a foe or something to avoid. Think about it. If you didn't feel awful about your using, would you have gotten sober? Pain most likely woke you up to recovery. Feeling deep emotional pain, then, was most likely very important in your decision to sober up.

In recovery we begin to feel a lot of feelings. With so many new feelings (because of new sober experiences), maybe you've tried to avoid uncomfortable feelings, or refrained from expressing them because you judge them in some way. Or, maybe you think you ought to be more mature about all your feelings.

DOI: 10.4324/9781003293231-10

Maybe you don't express your joy or pain, for whatever reason. Perhaps you stop yourself from crying, or getting angry, or laughing too loud. Or possibly, you feel so removed from feelings you don't even know what they are—or how you feel—and you want a definition you can understand.

What Are Feelings?

Here is one simple definition: **Feelings are the names we give *our own* felt experiences.**[1] Did you notice that *our own* is in italics?

Your feelings are what you experience in *your* thinking brain and feeling body.

My feelings are what I experience in my thinking brain and feeling body.

The Basics

The four basic feelings are sad, mad, glad, and afraid. Most likely, we all are familiar with these. I don't know about you, but I don't like feeling sad, mad, or afraid. I like feeling glad. There have been times I've listened to someone else tell me I should feel glad when I'm mad, and I've tried to do it. Listening to someone else tell me how I should feel has never made me feel glad, though. How about you?

Has anyone ever told you how you should or shouldn't feel? Or discounted your feelings in some other way? These people (the ones who want to convince you to feel something you don't) have a right to say whatever they want (yes, they really do), but remember:

It is up to you to know how you feel.

No one lives in your body but you. Only you can know how you feel. And all feelings are okay. Feelings just are. This is an important point, especially for those who wonder why they feel the way they do, or if their feelings are wrong or not acceptable in some way. Judging feelings is never helpful, no matter who is doing the judging.

As we mature, and certainly as we grow in recovery, we will experience more feelings than the basic four mentioned earlier. Feelings are nuanced and at times mixed. Sometimes sorting out an expanded Range of Feelings can be confusing and takes time. What is important when you are doing the sorting is to remember what is basic:

You always have permission to name your own feelings.

You are a human and this is your birthright. And you can take your time. In fact, taking the time to name your feelings is part of becoming an emotionally sober person. Yes, you might feel uncomfortable doing this because you will be sitting with your feelings, which may be new for you. If you try to will your feelings away or deny how you feel, however, they will persist, begging you to pay attention.

Any kind of denial of feelings is saying your feelings aren't important.

Are Feelings Important?

Yes, feelings are very important! There are more than a few good reasons why feelings are important in recovery.

One reason is that feelings help you know yourself. This may seem ridiculously simple and elementary, and maybe it is, but stick with me here. If you know yourself and how you feel about anything, you will know what you want and don't want, and what you like or dislike.

> **Knowing how you feel about things will help you know your innermost self so you can build and enjoy the life in recovery you want.**

If part of your recovery is to discover how to live a joyful drug-free life with meaning and purpose, the way to get there is to know YOU. And you do this by knowing how you feel about things.

Feelings Guide Our Yesses and No's

Your feelings will be the precursor to saying yes to what you want and no to what you don't want. In the best of cases, if something feels good, we say yes to it. If something doesn't feel good or right, we say no. For example, if you were cold and hungry you would say yes to a fresh hot meal but no to cold rotten leftovers. Spoiler alert: When it comes to people, though, we can get a little confused about what is good for us. The main idea here is that it is okay to trust your gut, whether with food, people, or anything else. Learning how to *feel* your gut, however, might take some time.

While sorting out feelings in early sobriety and over the life of recovery in general, sober people can get the yesses and no's mixed up. Reasons for this confusion around an authentic yes and no are often about some form of codependency or other family dysfunction, usually involving discounting of feelings (whether by oneself or others). **Chronic discounting of feelings can render us removed from knowing how we feel in our guts.**

With discounting in whatever form, some addicts have denied (not felt) their feelings for so long they don't know who they are. Therefore, inauthentic yesses and no's become habitual and so much a part of who they think they are because they have forgotten how they feel about things. Is this you?

Or some may secretly remember who they are but are too fearful to share their feelings and yesses and no's with anyone. They hide their true selves behind some version of a person they think acceptable. A person like this, we could say, is a person impersonating a person.

A Person Impersonating a Person?

Do you ever feel like you are a person impersonating a person? This may sound funny but is actually quite tragic. If you identify, have some compassion for yourself. If you know someone like this, a dose of compassion will help here, too.

As practicing addicts, many of us cut ourselves off from our feelings. By the time we sober up, many of us have had little or no ability to own and name our own feelings. Because of this, we couldn't express our true selves with others, even in sobriety.

The good news is that in recovery, we get to remember and discover who we are deep down inside our hearts and minds. We get to feel our feelings and then freely express ourselves to the world. This is how you can experience YOU in a substance-free body.

Be kind to yourself and others in your remembering, discovering, and sharing yourself with the world. You are YOU. You have your own feelings about things. You get to feel and share your yesses and no's.

Like a fortune cookie said: It is better to be an authentic version of yourself than a second-rate version of someone else.

If you are alive, though, you are still YOU, even if you feel like the great pretender. This means there is a place inside of you—and your heart—that feels. As said before, **all feelings are okay, and we all have permission to feel**. Taking this idea seriously may be your gateway into learning how to feel what is in your own gut and heart, so you can trust your gut and heart—with the ultimate goal of being able to freely express your true yesses and no's in relationships.

Whereas reacting emotionally codependent (eating and regurgitating spoiled food) may have been the norm, feeling feelings and acting rationally (reaching for fresh healthy food) will be a new way of relating to oneself and others. This will take practice over time. Think baby steps or small bites.

Denying Feelings Versus Honoring Feelings

As said before, in recovery, we may deny, avoid, or try to hide feelings. To do this is a recipe for depression, resentment, or relapse. To suppress feelings in sobriety can be done for a while, but eventually, deep, unfamiliar, and possibly scary feelings may surface. For those who have a history of any trauma, this may be especially true.

Note: Many addicted people have experienced various forms of trauma. This book does not explore trauma in detail. Healing from trauma may be beyond the scope of this book. Although the Twelve Step and other programs help heal, additional aid by mental health professionals can be of great benefit in understanding and working through deeper psychological and spiritual wounds.

Deep feelings may throw you off balance, but not to worry. If you learn to acknowledge your feelings as important, work through them, and you have support from other sober people or a mental health professional, you will be able to get through even the most painful of feelings. On the other side of the not-so-pleasurable (or really awful) feelings will be relief. Feelings come and go.

The Recovery Cycle reminds us that living drug free is a matter of being willing to experience a Range of Feelings, and that having feelings is okay and part of being human. **We are all human and therefore will experience many feelings, addict or not.**

Acknowledging feelings is to acknowledge our humanity.

By honoring your feelings, you honor you, your recovery, and being a part of the whole of humankind. So yes, again, feelings are very important.

Impulse Control and Naming Feelings

Because we are human, we have the capacity to name and describe our feelings with words. When we are afraid, we can say "I'm afraid." Then, we can talk about what we are afraid of and rationally see there is no Gila monster chasing us. Reptiles (like our Gila monster) and other animals do not have the ability of speech and largely react on instinct when they feel threatened and are afraid.

Addicts, too, like our animal brethren, have been known to react spontaneously on impulse when feeling threatened. This reacting does not come just in the form of using but in all areas of our lives and in our relationships, sometimes well into sobriety. Reacting doesn't typically yield positive outcomes, however. If we want positive results in our lives and relationships, we will want impulse control.

Impulse control is a hallmark of recovery.

Without impulse control in sobriety, we aren't pausing long enough to name our feelings. If we don't exercise some impulse control to name our feelings and make a positive decision, we are probably regressing to the fight-flight-freeze mode to protect ourselves.

Fight-Flight-Freeze

As you may know, the fight-flight-freeze response is the body's automatic, built-in mechanism to keep us safe from danger or harm. This means that when we are afraid (when our instincts are threatened because we think the Gila monster is at our heels), our bodies automatically take over to help protect us, while the rational thinking brain takes a break.

You may know what fight-flight-freeze looks like in the animal kingdom, but for the human animal in recovery, the picture is a bit different. Maybe you can relate to the following:[2]

Fight: Have you ever blown up at someone with mean words discharging out of your mouth, cruel words there to live forever in everyone's mind who was in earshot? Words you wished you could have taken back? Or have you ever attacked someone physically?

Flight: What about a time when you may have just plain avoided a situation and walked away seemingly unruffled, or nodded a cool yes when you knew you meant no? Or maybe you moved away to another country or hastily ended a perfectly good relationship, thinking greener pastures were out there somewhere?

Freeze: Perhaps there has been a moment when you froze, as if strange mouthless creature from another planet suddenly inhabited your body? Maybe you couldn't speak up for yourself because the alien inside you had a tight grip on your vocal cords, squeezing your self-esteem and spirit right out of you?

Whatever predominant style of emotional reacting you do (we typically gravitate to one but can resort to all three, depending on circumstances), it probably hasn't resulted in you being able to (in that moment) make a positive decision for yourself and your life.

In a highly emotional time, or if we are triggered in some way, it is almost impossible to pause, think rationally, work through feelings, and make a positive decision on our own behalf.

Under the Influence of Fear

For recovering people, we could call this impulsivity as being "under the influence of fear."

Reacting impulsively is kind of like being under the influence of your drug, with no ability to stop midstream. Have you ever felt you just had to finish your emotional binge, or that you couldn't control your behavior during an emotional time? Think about your last reactive emotional bender. Could you pause long enough to think about what you were afraid of?

In recovery, we learn to pause long enough to see that Gila monsters don't chase and kill, and unless you live in the southwestern United States or northern Mexico, they're nowhere around. Knowing monsters aren't chasing you, you can relax enough to pause and name your feelings, because after all: Recovery is about staying sober and living the good life we choose for ourselves. In other words:

> **We take the time to know how we feel about things so we can make positive decisions, rationally.**

If you want emotional sobriety in your life, learn to pause, clarify what you are feeling through your thinking brain, and name the feeling. Then you will be in a better position to make a positive decision that is good for you (so you can then act rationally rather than react emotionally).[3] This process of naming feelings is so crucial for emotional sobriety, I'll say it another way:

When we name our feelings, we can have a feeling-centered response as opposed to an emotionally-loaded reaction.

For sure, there are times when you won't need to pause, because you know how you feel and aren't afraid. The tool of pausing and naming feelings is a useful one, though, and can come in handy for all kinds of situations.

Fatima Practices Impulse Control, Naming Feelings, and Making a Positive Decision

"I went to visit my parents over the holidays. I felt anxious and afraid that I would want to drink. My mom told me, as she usually does, that I should lose weight and that she thought I should have chosen a career that would make me more money. I immediately wanted to tell her I was on a diet and defend my career. I wanted to yell at her, but I didn't. My stomach immediately hurt. I went to my room for a pause break. In my old room I realized I felt hurt and sad that my mom couldn't rejoice in my choices, and that my dad just sat there and didn't stick up for me. I felt afraid I wasn't good enough. I called my sponsor, which was a better decision than lashing out at my parents or stuffing my feelings. In talking to my sponsor, I realized I felt shamed and diminished. I am so glad I didn't fight with them or drink, though. I made a decision to stay in a hotel in the future so I could visit on my terms."[4]

Dry and High

For recovering people, if there is no pause or impulse control when we feel our emotions, especially when our instincts are threatened (because of fear), we may use again one day or make ourselves and/or others miserable in some emotionally reactive way.

Inadequate impulse control can manifest in unsavory, self-destructive behaviors like yelling at others, physically harming your spouse, over-exercising to the point of injury, flipping off other drivers on the highway, silently punishing your partner by smugly withholding something, seething with resentment and the like. This kind of emotional reactivity, with no honest introspection, is characteristic of what is known as a "dry drunk."

To be dry is to be in a perpetually negative emotional state, powered by a good dose of negative thinking. If you have experienced this, it is almost like a diseased evil monster is living inside your body eating away at your insides with its poison. To be monstrously dry is a way of getting high but without an outside substance. Haven't we all liked to get good and angry at times?

What Is a Dry Drunk?

A dry drunk is a person who is not using but hasn't made any internal changes. Instead of being genuinely satisfied with sobriety, the dry one acts like he is still serving a prison sentence. Others close to him may think it is almost harder to be around him than when he was using. Often, he has an astonishing lack of impulse control.

The emotional staples of the dry drunk are anger, resentment, and self-pity. Other shades of this dry existence are grandiosity or extreme inferiority, intolerance, being judgmental, and no ability for introspection. As you might imagine, it is no fun being around a dry drunk.

For sure, we all get emotional at times. We're human. No one is perfect. The point is to not make emotional reactivity (the dry way) your normal. It may feel familiar and comfortable but beware of getting stuck, enamored with your own reactive emotionality.

If you can pause when feeling emotional—and take a moment to name and work through your feelings—your chances of staying abstinent are better in the long term. Doing this, you will gain an ability to experience the gifts of recovery and the joy of being YOU. This is emotional sobriety. One good question to answer is: **Do you want sobriety or do you want so-DRY-ity?**

The "Questions to Help You Pause" exercise will help you develop an ability to pause, identify how you feel, and gain better perspective.

Questions to Help You Pause

Answer the following questions in writing.

1. Think about you before your sobriety.

    - Did you know how to name your feelings before recovery? Describe.
    - What did you do when feelings came up?
    - Did you consider the idea of working through your feelings? How?
    - How did you think about your feelings? Did you judge your feelings, or?
    - Did you ever consider how a feeling felt in your body? Describe.

2. Now think about your recovery.

    - Are you feeling anything now? What feeling is it?
    - Do you ever talk to anyone about how you are feeling? To who and how?

- Do you have an ability to ride the feeling out and let it pass? Or, if you avoid the feeling, what do you do to avoid the feeling, and what is the fear?
- Do you notice that feelings come and go? What is an example?
- Do you ever feel emotions in your body? Where?

Desensitizing to Feelings

For recovering people, feelings can be the most perplexing, uncomfortable, and scary part of sobriety. We all just want to feel good but (as you probably have guessed by now) that's just not realistic. We find all kinds of ways to avoid feelings, especially the yucky ones. Surprisingly, we even find ways to keep ourselves from feeling good, too, even though that is what we say we want.

My recovery became a lot easier when I learned to desensitize to my feelings. When I shared this with a sober friend, she said, "What does desensitization mean? Will I become less sensitive?"

Desensitization, I told my friend, means **getting used to experiencing uncomfortable feelings, with small-dose, incremental exposure to the thing that causes discomfort**. And desensitization doesn't mean becoming less sensitive, as my friend thought.

Desensitization actually means becoming increasingly sensitive as a person but in a positive way. You will gain a growing ability to tolerate and accept the good and not-so-good feelings. Feelings that used to be intolerable (such as embarrassment, anxiety, or shame) become bearable and sometimes useful in your sober journey. And, if you can sit with your own feelings and hold them gently, chances are you can be more open and accepting of the feelings of others. Simply put:

Desensitization to feelings means acquiring an increasing ability to accept an expanded Range of Feelings—yours and theirs.

This idea of desensitization isn't new. In the work of two behavior pioneers, psychologist Mary Cover Jones and psychiatrist Joseph Wolpe, desensitization means there will be a diminished emotional response with repeated exposure to the thing that causes fear, anxiety, or phobia.[5] More recently, author and psychotherapist Thom Rutledge expands on this idea of desensitization for addicts with his (acronym for fear) tool: Face it, Explore it, Accept it, Respond to it (FEAR).[6] This is the basis from which we launch into this idea of desensitizing to feelings in sobriety.

Note: As we discuss this idea of desensitization, keep in mind **those suffering from addiction—sober or not—are prone to all kinds of fears, and fear seems to be at the root of most emotional reactivity.**

With small-dose exposure to discomfort, the feelings are still there, but not overwhelming to the point of "I can't stand this!" (and I must react). With incremental desensitization, intense or uncomfortable feelings are experienced and mitigated by taking actions that ultimately result in:

I can feel my feelings, I can stand this, and I will be okay.

For example, let's say you need a job and are terrified of job interviews. The fear and anxiety are overwhelming. To desensitize to these feelings of fear and anxiety, you might do small-dose things like:

- Research how to do a job interview.
- Make a list of questions the interviewer might ask.
- Ask someone you know about their experience with interviews.
- Visualize going on an interview and seeing yourself as confident.
- Practice in front of a mirror.
- Do a mock interview with a friend, having your friend ask you questions.
- Pick out an interview outfit.
- Research the company before your interview.
- Get directions ahead of time to the interview place, making sure you will allow enough time to get there early.

With each of the aforementioned activities, you may notice an increasing ability to sit with any anxious or fearful feelings. The fear and anxiety are made less—in increments—with exposure to the topic of job interviews, and then specifically to your job interview.

The day of your interview, you might still feel some fear or anxiety, but the feelings will be manageable. You can stand it. You may also notice you have a measure of confidence. Because you have actively exposed yourself to job interview situations and information, you now have the skill of supervising your anxiety and so can sit with the mix of feelings. You may or may not get the job, but either way, the next interview or your first day on that job will be easier.

Is There a Reason I Don't Let Myself Feel Good?

Some recovering people manage to find a way to sabotage pleasure. This sense of being unworthy of feeling good often stems from a lack of self-esteem and the fear that accompanies low self-esteem. For a lot of sober people, this lack of self-esteem and fear are subconscious blocks to enjoying life. Feeling good (and loving themselves and others fully) may seem elusive and for other people.

In Twelve Step and other recovery programs, there are tools for becoming conscious of the blocks that keep recovering people from feeling good. Recovering people do the work, go through the pain of facing themselves or whatever they need to face, share with others, and feel better on the other side.

They grow and learn to feel good. **Recovering people upgrade their capacity to feel good.**

Some addicts, however, don't automatically do the work that will ultimately help them feel better and grow. The work of facing low self-esteem and accompanying fear may be too uncomfortable, even if a beautifully realized carrot (feeling good as YOU) is dangling at the end of the sober guide's elegant hand. Staying the same, longing for that carrot but never getting it, is comfortable and familiar. Some believe: *That carrot will never be mine,* or, *Carrots like that really don't exist.* Others, the more entitled ones, think: *The carrot is too far out of reach, you must bring it to me.*

It can be hard for recovering people to trust that carrots exist or are within reach. Instead, they become strangely attracted to what is familiar: Drama, Intensity, Pain, and Struggle (DIPS). Not so strange, though, if you think about it.

With our addictions, we were stuck on the merry-go-round prison. After sobering up, we got some relief, but the relief was short-lived with all the relationships and other life challenges we faced. The intense part of us needed the DIPS juice. Anything less seemed boring and flat, or weirdly uncomfortable.

So often our subconscious mind insists on old toxic patterns. Our addictive brains—even in recovery—seem to be wired for the DIPS. We could say some step off the merry-go-round and step on a wild and rickety roller coaster ride of ups and downs. This may be exciting but also a little precarious and unstable. Some like the scare and unpredictability, while others don't (who get stuck in pain). If you want off the roller coaster (or out of the pain), another ride awaits!

A magic carpet ride (which is what this entire book is about) can take you beyond the addiction theme park gates of limited thinking and being. This ride will take you to a grand, new land. You will be transported to the life you want.

If you want on that magic carpet, you must step off the roller coaster. Once you step on your magic carpet, you will soon be lifted and see beyond the addiction-themed walls of your self-constructed prison. As you transform, you will learn to be the seer who SEAS. This means you decide to Surrender with Equanimity, Acceptance, and Serenity (SEAS).

DIPS or SEAS?

Drama, Intensity, Pain, and Struggle do not have to be the norm just because you are an addict. Sometimes it may feel more exciting and juicier to be in the DIPS, and if that is what you want, go for it.

If you want out of the DIPS, however, here is something you can try:

Sit with your emotions, name your feelings, and then decide what you want to do or not do. In your decision-making, it might be

helpful to name your fears and get support. Ultimately, any decision is yours, but feedback from a trusted other is often helpful.
This other could be a sponsor, friend in your program, therapist, or
spiritual advisor.

We can't always bypass negative feelings, but we can always choose
how to sit and wiggle our way through them by deciding on something
positive to do or not to do and then follow up with that positive action
or inaction, respectively.

If you Surrender to this process of feeling enough times, Equanimity, Acceptance, and Serenity will become your new way of navigating
through life. You get to be the captain of you. Do you want to voyage
in choppy waters or calm seas?

Desensitizing to Pleasure

This idea of desensitizing to pleasure may sound puzzling because we all would
say we want to feel good, right? What is the reason we would need to desensitize to pleasure?

Believe it or not, as recovering people, it's easy to get used to feeling bad.
Some become workaholics. Others become obsessive worriers about the rela-
tives coming over, the children, the upcoming car purchase, what to plant in
the garden, or anything else. Still, others find a false sense of pleasure in their
secondary addictions, but then, the secondary addiction causes emotional pain.
And as said previously, many live in the DIPS in almost every situation. Feeling
bad can be a subconscious habit. Do you identify?

Often, we don't allow ourselves to experience pleasure that is good for us, as
if to enjoy life will always be something out of fairy tales. **In recovery, however,
we give ourselves permission to enjoy our lives and feel good.**

Accomplishing this, for some of us, will mean desensitizing to the discomfort we may feel while discovering pleasure and incorporating good feelings into our lives. This discomfort will be personal to each individual. One
friend of mine understands this concept as "desensitizing to the discomfort
of pleasure." I say:

> **Expect a learning curve as you desensitize to pleasure and to
> enjoying your life.**

Perhaps my own experience will shed some light on this.

When I sobered up years ago, I thought of all the things I wanted in life.
With these things, I thought, I would feel good all the time. In my mind, I
secretly manufactured a score of "if-onlys." If only I had this. If only I had that.
Then, I would get the if-only, and find myself complaining about some part of

it, or wanting something else. And then, voila! There would be yet another if-only, and I would feel dissatisfied all over again.

I revealed to a trusted friend this tendency. I expected my friend to say, "Make a gratitude list." My friend, however, said how difficult it had been for her to enjoy the good in her life and that she learned how to sit with her feelings of discomfort in meditation and in her day.

After that, I committed to a solid and consistent meditation practice. Soon, I recognized uneasy and anxious were my constant companions ever since I could remember. Any real joy I felt I had to hide away, like the M&Ms I used to secretly eat in a dark theater, well into sobriety.

I saw my thinking and beliefs were feeding the unease. It was no fun seeing my negative experience had nothing to do with life in the here and now, but instead, everything to do with my perceptions and projections, stemming from old rotten roots. My thinking was really screwy!

What had rooted in me was the idea that I was incomplete and a big, awkward mistake. Never enough "as is." Raised in an environment where I thought my only job was to be a show pony of a wicked sort, I turned into a performing seal for the world as an adult. My whole life, I never measured up. With this awareness, some very painful feelings came up. I let them come. Then they left, leaving room for good seed, the joy that is our birthright. And then the feelings would come again, and go again, too.

I slowly realized everything is an inside job and vigorously began taking responsibility for joy and actively appreciating when I felt good.

Now, if an "if-only" rears, I rein it in with some recovery tool—while honoring my feelings. With this comes cultivation of healthy pleasure and good feelings. What about you?

You might be thinking, *Sure, it's easy for you to say all this stuff about sitting through feelings and desensitization, you are decades sober and already have your good life.*

My response is: I have many feelings I still don't like. Embarrassment is my least favorite, next to anxiety and many other feelings we all feel. I'm still in the process of living a life of unlimited expansion, which includes risk, mistakes, successes, and feeling vulnerable. Still, I keep my Recovery Focus. And yes, my feelings of joy and capacity for pleasure have expanded too.

If you are confused about this idea of desensitizing to pleasure, think of it as the beginning of YOU growing and owning good feelings in you. As you do this, pay attention to anything in you that resists this, but keep wiggling toward your heaven and light anyway. Answering the questions in the "Planting Seeds for Growth" box may help you begin to do this. And, if you take some action in the "Growing Good Feelings" box you'll be on your way to cultivating your very own healthy pleasure. After all, as Carl Jung said:

> The knowledge of the heart is in no book and is not to be found in the mouth of any teacher, but grows out of you like the green seed from the dark earth.

Planting Seeds for Growth

If enjoying your life and feeling good is challenging for you, answer the following questions. Think of these questions as seeds you are planting in you to grow good feelings. Write out your answers. If you want to share your writing, do it with someone sober and trustworthy.

1. Is this idea of desensitizing to pleasure (or to the discomfort of pleasure) a new concept? How do you understand this idea?
2. Do you feel challenged by this idea of desensitizing to pleasure? If so, what is challenging?
3. Do you ever notice any unruly negative thinking? Do you believe negative thinking might be a way to keep you from feeling good? Explain.
4. Where do you think your negative thoughts come from? Explain. If this question feels it might be too upsetting for you, skip it and seek professional help or get help from your trusted sober guide.
5. Do you notice when you feel good? How do you appreciate those feel-good times?
6. Is it easy for you to express your joy? If no, what gets in the way?
7. How do you know when you are feeling good and joyful? Explain.
8. However long you are sober, do you think you are worthy of feeling good? Why or why not?

Growing Good Feelings

Here are a few ideas about how you can grow some good feelings and move toward good, healthy pleasure:

• Discover what you like to do and do it. Do you like to play cards? Read? Go to museums?
• Make it a priority to do what you like to do. Do it more than once.
• If you like animals, pet a dog or a cat and notice how you feel when you are doing it. Or go to a petting zoo.
• Spend time with a friend you feel good around.
• Talk to a trusted person about how you want to learn how to feel better. Ask them what they do to feel good.

- Play your favorite music.
- Write a thoughtful letter to someone you care about, telling them specifically what you appreciate about them.
- Dance alone to music you like.
- If you are with someone you like, tell them what you like about them.
- Take a walk in nature.

These are just a few of ideas, but you get the gist. They are simple things. Choose some simple activity that feels good to you and do it. If it feels uncomfortable, that's okay. This is how we desensitize and lean into healthy pleasure. Build your joy. Notice the pleasure and good feelings grow. You have a right to feel good because:

Recovery includes feeling good.[7]

More Ways to Experience Feelings

In addition to desensitization, there are other ways you can learn to experience a Range of Feelings. You might have an easier recovery if you can:

- Experience emotions and name your feelings.
- Refrain from judging your feelings.
- Realize feelings come and go.
- Understand feelings don't kill.
- Recognize feelings are not facts.
- Share feelings with a trusted sober person.
- Develop a sense of self-compassion for your feelings.

Too Much Emphasis on Feelings?

This is not too much emphasis on feelings. Firstly, this chapter is about the "Range of Feelings" part of the cycle. Some attention to this very important part of recovery—of life—needs to be addressed. This part of the Recovery Cycle emphasizes that we acknowledge, honor, and experience our feelings. With this acceptance, feelings flow, come, and go.

Too much focus on feelings, however, and doing nothing but continuing to focus on how bad we feel is not a good thing. This can be addictive. With extended focus on the not-so-good feelings, the tendency to case-build (i.e., find things to support our bad feelings about ourselves, others, and the world) may result. This leads to more negative feelings and self-pity, which ultimately translates into a "poor me" state of mind. Also, spending too much time trying to figure out why we feel the way we do can be just as much of a downer.

Staying stuck focusing on feelings is like paying too much attention to the weather and analyzing why Mother Nature is making it rain on your wedding day. It doesn't do any good to try and figure Mother Nature out. Mother Nature does what she does, and rain comes and goes according to her laws. She can't be controlled. The feeling experience can be assuaged by moving the wedding ceremony indoors, or changing the venue, or putting up a tarp. The question is, what experience do you want on your wedding day or any other day? Yes, it may be a bummer to get rained out, and disappointment understandable, but what would be a positive decision that would help you accept the circumstances as is? It could be that a change in attitude is the answer.

Choosing Guides

By giving feelings proper respect, it is relatively simple to put the focus back on recovery. Ideally, especially in early recovery, you have enlisted someone who listens to you and can guide you when you experience feelings. You may have found this person at a Twelve Step or another recovery group. This someone, if you've chosen well, will point you in the direction of emotionally sober recovery. **This guide doesn't judge you or your feelings and supports you in taking action to work through your emotions.** If your feelings become debilitating, or you've experienced any trauma, you may want to go to a mental health professional as well. This goes for everyone, including therapists.

A Word About Guidance—This Is Super Important!

The best guide for an addict in the sober journey is nonjudgmental and has no investment in the addict's decisions.

The relationship is about supporting the recovering person's journey, not about the decision or choice itself.

With this, the recoverer can take responsibility for who they want to be and will learn to make decisions based on what is in their own mind and heart.

Many people in recovery know we can move on from negative feelings with the satisfaction of staying the sober course. They also know sharing good feelings can grow more good feelings. If you listened to your feelings when choosing your guide, ideally your guide will be just right for you. Sometimes we pick someone who might not be the right fit initially. We can always find another someone who is better suited, however.

This guide may know if you are too focused on your feelings or if you have gone the opposite way and don't know how you feel about anything. This may be especially true for those new in recovery. Your guide will help support you through your feelings and embrace your drug-free life of infinite expansion and love. **Having someone with whom you share honestly is vital.** This can't be stressed enough—if you don't have someone like this, pick someone. This person will help your recovery be easier. **This person is not an all-knowing God but a fellow human being like you.**

And, if you believe in a Higher Power or something greater than you (i.e., if you have any spiritual belief), this will be a place you can turn for support as well. Many new in recovery (especially in Twelve Step programs) have found both consulting with other sober people and a relationship with a Higher Power is the best combination for working through feelings.

We do all this feeling stuff knowing other sober people are doing it with us. No more being alone with feelings. No more doing recovery alone. With others, recovery is simpler and easier.

This way of learning to work through and accept an expanded Range of Feelings is how we can ultimately focus back on recovery. With a greater acceptance of feelings, we understand ourselves and each other better. Hence, our vision of the recovery we want for ourselves becomes even more clear.

What you have read so far completes a basic explanation of the Recovery Cycle. Pretty simple so far, right? The next chapter is about weighing the cost factor of any decision, not just about using. We will see how this tool can be practical, spiritual, and transformative.

Recovery Recap

- A Range of Feelings means you will feel a lot of feelings in recovery: some pleasurable, some painful, and many in between.
- Mad, sad, glad, and afraid are the basic four feelings.
- You have permission to name your own feelings.
- Knowing how you feel about things will help you know your innermost self so you can build and enjoy the life you want.
- Feelings help you know yourself and are the precursors to your yesses and no's. Feelings are what make you YOU.
- It is up to you to know how you feel.
- Impulse control is a hallmark of recovery.
- Taking the time to name your feelings increases your chances of acting positively on your own behalf.
- Desensitization means getting used to uncomfortable feelings by way of small-dose exposure to the thing that causes discomfort.
- You can grow good feelings.
- An overfocus on the not-so-good feelings can lead to self-pity and a "poor me" state of mind.

- We learn to experience, acknowledge, honor, and accept feelings with the help of other sober people.
- Find help where you don't feel judged. This help comes from people in recovery, sponsors, spiritual guides, and/or mental health professionals.
- By working through feelings in the way this chapter outlines, your vision of the recovery you want for yourself will become even more clear.

Clinician's Corner

A good guide creates a safe therapeutic space by allowing all emotions to be, where all feelings can be shared without the threat of judgment or criticism. Do you allow yourself to be, feel, think, and share honestly in the presence of a trusted other, now that you've given up that something for the duration of this book?

Owning your own stuff will help you support others through painful feelings as well as grow more pleasurable ones. As usual, answer the questions (in the FEEL exercise) before giving them to your client.

FEEL Exercise—Foster Effective Emotion Labeling (30–60 Minutes)

Write out your answers.

1. Describe your understanding of a "Range of Feelings."
2. Do you have a safe person with whom you can share all your feelings? If yes, how did you come to believe this person was a safe place for you? If you don't have this person, what prevents you from finding someone?
3. Do you have an ability to say "yes" to what you want and "no" to what you don't want? If not, what prevents you from doing so? If there is fear, what are you afraid of? Or, do any other feelings come up when you think about this?
4. Share your findings with your therapist or sober guide. If this feels too risky or scary, discuss your fear (or anything else you relate to in this chapter) with a safe someone.
5. Google a feelings wheel and review it. How are you feeling right now?
6. Extra Credit: Go back to the exercises "Questions to Help You Pause" and "Planting Seeds for Growth" in this chapter. Write out your answers.

Straight Shot (3–5 Minutes)

1. What are the four basic feelings (as stated in this chapter)? Describe which of the four you are feeling right now and write about it with the who, where, what, and when.

Notes

1. Antonio Damasio, *Self Comes to Mind: Constructing the Conscious Brain* (New York: Random House, 2012), 116–118; Antonio Damasio, *Feeling and Knowing: Making Minds Conscious* (New York: Random House, 2021), 78–79. Damasio's view, in very simple terms, says feelings are mental associations that are linked to a physical (emotional) response we experience in our bodies. Basically, this means feelings and emotions are different, but they are linked. Mostly in the colloquial world, the terms feelings and emotions are used interchangeably. To keep it simple, I've opted to use the word *feelings* to describe feelings and what many think of as emotions.
2. I've described in a light brush stroke what fight-flight-freeze behavior might look like here, but there are physical symptoms as well, which are also clues you might not feel safe. For anyone who has experienced any trauma, fight-flight-freeze may be all too familiar and may indicate posttraumatic stress disorder. This book does not cover the scope of trauma that is known to many recovering people. For a list of physical symptoms of the fight-flight-freeze response and more on trauma, see "Fight, Flight, Freeze Responses," Manitoba Trauma Information & Education Centre, accessed December 20, 2021, https://trauma-recovery.ca/impact-effects-of-trauma/fight-flight-freeze-responses/.
3. Following up with action that backs a positive decision is key to emotional sobriety, growth in recovery, and to working through feelings we might consider negative. Pat Allen has said numerous times in her Want® Trainings, "The way out of a negative feeling is a positive decision followed by action or inaction, ASAP."
4. This sharing of life stories and feelings has a palliative effect on the sharer whose feelings may have been discounted in childhood. For additional reading on this idea of naming feelings, read Daniel J. Siegel and Tina Payne Bryson, *The Whole Brain Child: 12 Revolutionary Strategies to Nurture Your Child's Developing Mind* (New York: Bantam, 2012), 27–36. This book (for parents) describes how we can integrate the right and left hemispheres of our brains and calm big emotions by telling stories and naming our feelings; Siegel says, "Name it to tame it."

5. "Profile: Mary Cover Jones," *Psychology's Feminist Voices*, accessed December 20, 2021, https://feministvoices.com/profiles/mary-cover-jones; Russell A. Dewey, "Desensitization and Exposure Therapies," in *Psychology: An Introduction* (2017–2018 rev.), www.psywww.com/intropsych/ch13-therapies/desensitization-and-exposure-therapies.html. Mary Cover Jones is most known for a study in which she treated three-year-old Peter's "fear of a white rabbit with a variety of fear-reducing procedures. The most successful procedure was that of 'direct conditioning,' in which a pleasant stimulus (food) was presented simultaneously with the rabbit. As the rabbit was gradually brought closer to him in the presence of his favorite food, Peter grew more tolerant, and was able to touch it without fear." Joseph Wolpe is known for "systematic desensitization." This therapeutic technique assumes that what has been learned (conditioned) can be unlearned by incorporating relaxation techniques along with exposure of the thing that causes anxiety or phobia.

6. Thom Rutledge, *Embracing Fear: How to Turn What Scares Us Into Our Greatest Gift* (New York: HarperCollins, 2002), 15.

7. Patrick Carnes, *A Gentle Path Through the Twelve Steps: The Classic Guide for All People in the Process of Recovery* (Center City, MN: Hazelden, 2012), 61; Rick Hanson, *Hardwiring Happiness: The New Brain Science of Contentment, Calm and Confidence* (New York: Random House, 2013). "Growing Good Feelings" is a close cousin to the "Gentleness Break" in Carnes. This Gentleness Break is about rewarding oneself after completing the work of a very thorough First Step (presented in his book). Recovering people must learn to reward themselves with some gentle, feel-good parts of life not only to foster healthy pleasure after some rigorous step work, but also to achieve more balance in life. Learning how to incorporate some gentleness and good feelings into all the difficult, personal work of recovery is a way to integrate more balance, comfort, and ease into the life of the recovering person. Hanson's is another book to check out to increase joy. This resource, using the acronym HEAL, offers a simple method to build new neural pathways to increase positive emotions.

Works Cited

Carnes, Patrick. *A Gentle Path Through the Twelve Steps: The Classic Guide for All People in the Process of Recovery*. Center City, MN: Hazelden, 2012.

Damasio, Antonio. *Self Comes to Mind: Constructing the Conscious Brain*. New York: Random House, 2012.

Damasio, Antonio. *Feeling and Knowing: Making Minds Conscious*. New York: Random House, 2021.

Dewey, Russell A. "Desensitization and Exposure Therapies." In *Psychology: An Introduction* (2017–2018 rev.). www.psywww.com/intropsych/ch13-therapies/desensitization-and-exposure-therapies.html.

Hanson, Rick. *Hardwiring Happiness: The New Brain Science of Contentment, Calm and Confidence*. New York: Random House, 2013.

Manitoba Trauma Information & Education Centre. "Fight, Flight, Freeze Responses." Accessed December 20, 2021. https://trauma-recovery.ca/impact-effects-of-trauma/fight-flight-freeze-responses/.

"Profile: Mary Cover Jones." *Psychology's Feminist Voices*. Accessed December 20, 2021. https://feministvoices.com/profiles/mary-cover-jones

Rutledge, Thom. *Embracing Fear: How to Turn What Scares Us Into Our Greatest Gift*. New York: HarperCollins, 2002.

Siegel, Daniel J., and Tina Payne Bryson. *The Whole Brain Child: 12 Revolutionary Strategies to Nurture Your Child's Developing Mind*. New York: Bantam Books, 2012.

8   Prices and Prizes

In This Chapter

- What Are Prices and Prizes?
- Weigh It to Sway It
- Gratification Versus Satisfaction: You Choose
- Secondary Addictions

Active addiction robs addicts of choice. In recovery, though, choices abound. Deciding how to live and love best in recovery proves to be a baffling, exciting, and tall order for many recovering people. Addicts can make themselves downright crazy with so many choices! This chapter presents a simple tool to help with choices and decision-making: Prices and Prizes.

What Are Prices and Prizes?

A Price is the downside or cost factor for any choice. A Price for using, for example, might be the dissolution of your marriage, jail time, or death. When using, rarely did any of us think about the highest possible Price.

A Prize is the upside or benefit for any choice. It's kind of like a reward. The Prize for using might be feeling good or numbing pain. The Prizes for using seduce addicts into using more and more.

Prices and Prizes are about more than using, though.

Choices Galore

There are many choices beyond using. This becomes more obvious the longer we are in recovery. First, we realize we are no longer victims of our addictions. Then, we come to realize we have choices in so many things. Our lives become filled with choices. Sometimes we have a difficult time making a choice. This could be something important like who to marry or something minor like what vegetable to order for your dinner side.

With so many choices, big and little, making a decision can become paralyzing. It seems too many options gum up our decision-making process, sometimes

DOI: 10.4324/9781003293231-11

to the point of not making any choice. Or, with so many options, we often become less, not more, satisfied with our choice.[1] Basically, too many choices can make us nuts!

Rumination

Even with just a few choices, we can make ourselves literally sick in our bodies with extended ruminating. If you were to go online and look up "stress" and "rumination," you would find articles and studies that point to rumination as a threat to physical and mental health, due to the elevated cortisol levels rumination induces. Also, some research links rumination to depression. But instead of going online for evidence of the ill effects of rumination and cortisol, think of a time when you have ruminated and how it felt in your body. If you don't know what I'm talking about, keep reading.

Rumination is the think/feel loop. This is when we go from thinking about something to feeling, then back to thinking about the same thing, and then back to feeling. This think/feel loop can go on and on. When no positive decision is made—followed by action—the think/feel loop can loop tirelessly and endlessly.

We loop-de-loop because we want to make the best choice. We think we are solving the problem by thinking about it. We think there is the perfect choice, maybe even the choice God wants for us: the choice that is the right choice.

Rumination can cause stress. The thought that there is a preordained right choice adds to the stress. Sometimes we forget that for many things, there is just no right choice.

So much of being human is in not knowing what the future holds with the choices and decisions we make. Knowing this doesn't always help with the rumination problem though. **Recovery becomes a lot easier when we can use a concrete tool to help us get out of ruminating and into action.**

One tool to get out of the rumination mire is Prices and Prizes.

Weigh It to Sway It

With Prices and Prizes, we are reminded that at any moment in time we can deliberately and thoughtfully consider many sides of any choice or decision; thus, we begin to get out of rumination. Because extended rumination can create havoc in the addictive brain and a big stall in your life, the importance of weighing Prices and Prizes throughout our lives can't be stressed enough.

> **Evaluating Prices and Prizes helps you choose what is best for your recovery and life.**

The ideal is to sway a decision in favor of the life YOU want. Weighing Prices and Prizes can get you out of the dizzying rumination loop. This is an easy thing to do. Doing it is the beginning of YOU considering your choices. Just taking the action of weighing the cost for any choice gets us closer to the relief of making the decision. This consideration of Prices and Prizes is a simple thing to do.

The easiest way to weigh Prices and Prizes is to simply consider the highest Price of any choice. For example, take any choice you have right now. Pick anything. Now, consider the worst-case scenario if you make that choice. Then ask yourself if you are willing to live with that outcome, or in other words, pay the highest possible Price.

If you still can't decide, the more thorough way is to consider both the Prices and Prizes. For instance, let's say you have a choice about whether or not to take a new job. First, you would gather all the information you could about that job. Then you would identify the upsides, or Prizes. Let's say for this job, the biggest Prize for you is the great salary.

Now, name the downsides, or Prices. A huge downside, or the highest Price, you decide, is a 120-mile-a-day commute.

Next, look at both the Prices and Prizes and see if you can live with the highest possible Price. Perhaps even though the salary is great, you know too well this could mean a two-hour commute each way on a bad day. Driving that much time in traffic won't work for you. That is your bottom line.

Someone else may be willing to do the drive, by the way. You know this because you've asked all your friends what they would do, and one friend said she'd take the job in a minute, even with the commute. Your friend's response is one reason why choices can be so difficult—the opinions of others can muddy your own. But remember:

Your choices are individual and up to YOU. What is good for you
may be horrible for someone else, and vice versa.

If you want more help with this, do the exercise in the "How to Choose with Prices and Prizes" box.

How to Choose with Prices and Prizes

Do you have a choice or decision to make about something right now? If yes, here is a way you can make your decision:

1. Gather all the information about your choice.
2. Write out all the Prizes, or upsides.
3. Write out the Prices, or downsides.
4. Determine the highest possible Price.
5. If you are unsure about the highest Price, ask someone you respect, or your guide, to give you feedback. (Because our addict brains are

great at rationalizing, we sometimes can't identify the highest possible Price. This is where good, honest feedback can help.)
6.   Ask yourself if you are willing to pay the highest possible Price.
7.   Make the choice and follow up with action to back up your decision.

If you are willing to pay the highest possible Price, then maybe you will go for it. This means you will take responsibility for your decision if you end up having to pay that highest Price. Basically, you have decided you can live with the consequences of your decision.

If you aren't willing to pay the highest Price tag, then maybe you won't go for it. You don't want the gamble. You, too, have decided you can live with the consequences of your decision.

Some choices are multifaceted and just aren't that easy. With difficult decisions, it might be wise to get counsel from someone who can be objective. Being able to talk it out can be helpful in determining more Prices and Prizes; and with the freedom to share, different choices just might emerge. Choices you hadn't considered. A thoughtful discussion about Prices and Prizes—and choices—can be a creative event.

Some choices are just not that easy, but using the tool of Prices and Prizes gives us more clarity around choices and about what we want and don't want. The most important part is taking some action (and responsibility) around difficult decisions. Even polling friends is an action. Just know that the polling is gathering data for you to ultimately make the choice that is right for YOU. Prices and Prizes are about what YOU can personally live with.

What If I Make a Mistake?

With some choices, after all the sampling, information gathering, and the Price/Prize review, making your choice may be a leap of faith. Sometimes we might look back and wish we'd made a different choice. The good news about these less favorable outcomes—what some might call mistakes—is there is always a lesson. So, there is a silver lining with decisions we make that don't turn out like we would have wished. That Prize? As one of my mentors said, we grow in wisdom and grace. **It's okay to make mistakes.**[2] It really is. That's how we learn.

Gratification Versus Satisfaction: You Choose

Once we have a choice about using and choose to stay sober, a world of choices opens up. While using, choices are limited and centered around the addiction. Choices such as what dealer to visit or how to avoid too many repeat visits to the corner liquor store, dessert shop, or massage parlor rob addicts of precious time and energy. These choices keep addiction sufferers from living a satisfied life. Gratification through our drug was the aim. After sobering up, though, choices are endless. You always have a choice. One choice is: Do you want to live a gratified life or a satisfied life?

A Gratified Lifestyle

If your answer is a gratified life, that is your prerogative, but beware: What this means is that pleasure is your primary aim, which is fine. The cost factor, however, according to one empirical study on three distinct routes to happiness (i.e., pleasure, engagement, and meaning), indicates you might miss out on a fuller life with the sole pursuit of pleasure.[3]

Choices of a gratified lifestyle often include the primary addiction, but not always. Secondary addictions often crop up after getting sober, and these may feel pleasurable for sure, but there will be a cost. **There is a cost for every choice**.

Some sober people live lives of gratification and switch one addiction for another, such as overeating or over consumerism in place of alcoholism. The Prize for this kind of gratification may be avoidance of pain. Sadly though, this secondary addiction, if not acknowledged and dealt with, can become a part of this addict's life, and pain will be locked—maybe forever—in the depths of his soul. This may sound melodramatic, but this seems to be the way it is with us addicts.

Other forms of gratification come in the form of blaming others, putting others down, gossip, button-pushing, or any behaviors that lend themselves to feeling good at the expense of another. We all may have been guilty of this conduct, but if this is the norm without misgivings and action to do better, genuine satisfaction will be dim.

In a gratified lifestyle, both secondary addictions and an "I'm better than you" mentality escalate typically to avoid underlying pain. With either orientation, satisfaction will be transient or maybe even nonexistent. Gratification prevails at the expense of the addict's seemingly lost essential nature (his original sense of wholeness).

Some addicts who are gratification junkies may have convinced themselves all is good and behave in ways to keep the pain hidden. On the outside, all may appear fine. The pain may even be hidden from themselves. This is denial. The addict within is sly, seductive, and powerful. It often ploys deep in the subconscious mind. For those who choose a gratified lifestyle, know that secondary addictions, power plays, and denial are the tools for existing in a scary world.

What Is Denial?

Denial is a refusal to acknowledge the reality or fact that a painful event, thought, or feeling exists.

Denial can protect one's psychological well-being in traumatic situations or any situation that produces anxiety or conflict, past or present. It is one of the most primitive defense mechanisms.

A Satisfied Life

For addicts who want to live a satisfied life, there is a willingness to experience both pleasure and pain—a Range of Feelings—in exchange for transcendence. **A satisfied life in recovery means life is acceptable with all the ups and downs**. Pain may not be enjoyed (who enjoys pain?), but working through whatever needs attention is accepted while knowing pain will pass. The discomfort of working through the pain is a Price. **Feeling good is important and appreciated, but not to the point of denying pain or problems**.

This satisfied life is promoted by a faith that all is well, without a Pollyanna facelift. The satisfaction of making it through problems, along with a never-ending blossoming of one's SELF (original sense of wholeness), is the Prize. A bonus Prize is faith increases while love grows and deepens. All of this means one has an overall sense of well-being. This is a satisfied life.

Well-Being = "A Good or Satisfactory Condition or Existence[4]

For anyone out there who thinks good or satisfactory is scoff-worthy (I know someone who pooh-poohed this idea of satisfactory), think about the ups and downs of life—we all have them. If we have an expectation that each moment will be blissful, fantastic, or even happy, we are fooling ourselves and setting ourselves up for a big disappointment.

I especially like the word satisfactory because it implies a balanced, even, accepting state. Satisfactory, in a simple and progressively easier recovery, means you can have an extraordinary life, full of a lot of exciting things, but in general, you have an ability to be satisfied, even in the most trying situations.

Do you think well-being is a choice we make for ourselves?

So, which do you want? A satisfied life or a gratified life? We all have choices, choices in everything, in every moment.

If you are in a battle in your own mind about satisfaction versus gratification, or anything else, the rest of your day or life could depend on what choice you make today and what you DO with that choice.

Secondary Addictions

If you choose a satisfied life but aren't ready to give up your secondary addiction, that's okay. But be conscious of this: You might be avoiding something if you need something addictively. **The pleasure of the secondary addiction outweighs sitting with some emotional pain.** What we often avoid is some uncomfortable truth about ourselves. That's been my experience.

I smoked cigarettes the first five years of my sobriety and overate for the first 10 or so. A pack of gold Marlboros and a big plate of anything dripping with gobs of hot melted cheese were my best friends. Frozen yogurt every night was a staple, too. At some point during that first five years, I sensed there was some pain I was avoiding, but I just didn't want to quit smoking. Then one day, I became ready to sit through painful feelings (i.e., to get out of denial) without cigarettes, and I quit cold turkey. It was harder than quitting drinking.

Then, over the next five years, I dealt with my overeating problem. This choice led me to dealing with buried wounds from my past. I became very rigid about food for a while, which I discovered was just another way of trying to control my emotions. Eventually, over some time and with good support, I got help, desensitized to feeling some gnarly emotions, and the food problem slowly went away. Pizza and all cheesy things quit singing to me. I don't have any problems with food anymore at all. Really. Food is a nonissue. For us overeaters, we know this is truly a miracle.

The point about all this is, don't be surprised if a secondary addiction perks up. Just be aware that you have a choice to deal with it or not. And if you choose not to deal with it, know you may be avoiding something. Know you may be making the choice to gratify yourself or self-soothe with your secondary addiction. Know this secondary addiction could be harmful to your body, relationships, or soul. If this is your choice, enjoy the secondary addiction, but be kind to yourself. If we choose to consciously engage in a secondary addiction, we may still live a satisfied life.

To live a satisfied life depends on conscious intention.

I know a colleague, also an overeater and alcoholic, who was in a tremendous amount of stress while her husband was dying. Her doctor told her to overeat because she seemed to be close to losing her sanity and sobriety. She overate with the consciousness of why she was doing it. She knew she would gain weight, and she was willing to pay that Price. This is how she chose to handle her stress. After her husband died, she went back to normal eating and lost the weight. She did this and felt satisfied and okay with it. This woman lives a satisfied life.

Another sober person I know said he has realized his recent online shopping excursions had everything to do with managing uncomfortable feelings around an employment situation. He said it was a way for him to feel some comfort, but he knew it wasn't the solution to his problem. He was conscious of the discomfort, talking to his guide about it, and working on the employment issue in a way he could, all at the same time. This man lives a satisfied life because of his conscious intention.

Balance and Imbalance

Addicts seem to be prone to imbalances. After sobering up, we eat too much or become highly rigid in our diets. We become workaholics or procrastinate in finding work. We don't ever say what is bothering us or inevitably weave our woes into any and every conversation. Do you identify?

Some think that taming the crazies will make them boring. Unfortunately, these addicts may continue to be at the whim of denial. Until we find a way to balance out the imbalances—add discipline and structure to where there once was little—our lives may stay lopsided in ways harmful to our well-being and maybe even the well-being of others. Denial can win if we believe, "I'm an addict and I don't have control over my addictive nature." Some think the imbalances are funny.

In psychological terms, this laughing at our own pain can be referred to colloquially as the "gallows laugh."[5] We are essentially laughing at our own destruction when we laugh off our destructive imbalances. Moreover, with this laughing, we can con others into laughing with us; this in turn endorses the self-destruct mode. This kind of reinforcing gallows laughter can insure continued helplessness around any addiction.

Think of the person who shares at a meeting that he binged on a gallon of ice cream the night before and then jokingly says, "This is what we do." Or the girl who over-exercises to the point of needing hip replacement surgery and says, "It's a good thing I can get a hip replacement because I'm probably going to need two or three!" She may laugh, and get others to laugh with her, but at what cost?

The point of this? Be mindful of your imbalances and know the cost factor. Sure, we may laugh in identification and have a sense of humor about ourselves. Laughter is healing, for sure, but if our game is to talk and act as if we are helpless, hapless human beings without any solutions for our imbalances, we might as well expect to be chronically imbalanced. This is okay, if you are willing to pay the price. Just know:

**Imbalances may indicate you may be avoiding something,
such as feelings, or that you are buying into old unsupportive
beliefs about yourself.**

(These negative beliefs about yourself can be a major cause of not feeling good, by the way.)

I don't subscribe to the notion that recovering addicts are irrevocably bent toward a life of imbalance. I just don't. I've witnessed addicts move from wild disparities to an even state of mind and body. And incidentally, the people I'm thinking of are not boring people. They all wrestled with what they wanted for themselves in recovery and made a choice, and then a lot of other choices along the way. Then, these people followed up with positive action.

Choice gives us an opportunity to decide what is important to us. **Making a positive decision about something—and then doing it—is where we find the freedom to be ourselves in our own way**. So, if we say our choice is balance, harmony, or anything else, what then are we doing to demonstrate that? In the doing is where a Price is paid, however.

For example, let's say I want to have a healthy body so I can enjoy my life more. This will require more balance in my exercise program. So, am I scaling back or upping my exercise to something reasonable? Have I consulted with others to figure out what is reasonable? Am I then doing what is reasonable and being accountable to someone about how much I am exercising?

Breaking any habit around an imbalance (in this case, no exercise or over-exercising) will probably feel uncomfortable. The discomfort I feel around changing up my routine and becoming accountable with support is part of the Price of more balance with my exercise routine. With this, I am congruent with what I say I want—a healthier body so I can enjoy my life—and I am paying the Price to get it *by doing something.*

> **Little by little balance can become the new norm—if this is what**
> **you want and are willing to pay the Price—and enjoy the Prize.**

When we can pause, make thoughtful decisions, and follow up with action, we are closer to finding balance and harmony in our lives. This emerges one transaction at a time.

We are now prepared to move on and look at the Recovery Cycle with a few real-life examples. In the next chapter, you will meet Gerry and Sissy. We will see how they use the tools of Prices and Prizes and transform as they move through the Recovery Cycle.

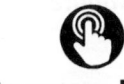

Recovery Recap

- We have many choices beyond using in recovery.
- Rumination causes stress—we can make ourselves crazy and physically ill with extended ruminating.
- A Price is the downside or cost factor for any choice. A Prize is the upside or benefit for any choice.
- Evaluating Prices and Prizes allows you to choose in a timely way what is best for your recovery and life.
- You have a choice about living a gratified life (where pleasure is your primary aim) or a satisfied life (where you are willing to experience both pleasure and pain for transcendence and for an overall sense of well-being).
- Imbalances may indicate you may be avoiding something, such as feelings, or that you are buying into old unsupportive beliefs about yourself.
- To live a satisfied life depends on conscious intention.
- Secondary addictions are often in response to buried emotional pain and manifest in imbalances.
- More balance in recovery is possible—if you are willing to pay the Price.

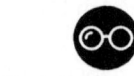

Clinician's Corner

You've probably noticed that societal, parental, and other relational influencers (maybe even some on social media) inevitably weigh in on what your client should or should not do. These opinions in your client's headroom proliferate and can inhibit differentiation, individuation, and actualization (á la Bowen, Jung, and Maslow, respectively).

Any good therapist knows it is not our job to opine about a client's choice or make decisions clients can make for themselves. We may think we have the right answers, but we don't. We guide with an accepting presence. Your task then, as a clinician, will be in helping clients find their own answers so they may be *themselves* and live the life *they* want. The following exercise is one way to assist clients in their own decision-making process and maturation.

As usual, you do the exercise, too. Also, Number 1 is especially helpful in a group setting, written out on a whiteboard or oversized wall Post-It, using a client's real example in front of the group.

What Do YOU Want? (25–45 Minutes)

Write out the answers.

1. Write out a decision/choice you have that you haven't decided on yet. It can be anything big or small. Then underneath make two columns opposite each other; write the word "Prices" for one column and "Prizes" for the other.

    Now fill in the Prices and Prizes for your potential decision. If it is a big decision, get help with coming up with the highest Price. (If you want to see an example of this exercise, skip ahead and see Gerry's examples in the next chapter.)
    After writing your list, are you more clear about what to do or not do? If not, get help from someone you respect and discuss your writing.

2. Do you think you have a secondary addiction or have an imbalance in some area? If yes, what do you think you might be avoiding? What old belief is preventing you from dealing with your secondary addiction? Do you want to give up your secondary addiction? Why or why not? What feelings do you think would surface?

3. Using your own experience, describe your understanding of a life of gratification and a satisfied life. Which do you want and why? How are you living either at this time?

Straight Shot (5–10 Minutes)

1. Write out the Prices and Prizes for using/acting out.
2. Do you have a secondary addiction? If yes, are you okay with it and why?

Notes

1. Sheena S. Iyengar and Mark R. Lepper, "When Choice Is Demotivating: Can One Desire Too Much of a Good Thing?" *Journal of Personality and Social Psychology* 79, no. 6 (2000): 995–1006, https://doi.org/10.1037/0022-3514.79.6.995. This fun and often-cited study showed that "people are more likely to purchase gourmet jams . . . when offered a limited array of 6 choices rather than a more extensive array of 24 or 30 choices." Have you ever experienced the paralysis of having too many choices?
2. Recovering Couples Anonymous, *A Twelve Step Program for Couples*, 4th ed. (Oakland, CA: World Service Organization for Recovering Couples Anonymous, 2011), 55. This statement, "It is OK to make mistakes," is one of the "Safety Guidelines" in the book. Although written for couples to help foster intimacy and better communication, this statement applies for any choice we make, as well, and for life in general!
3. Christopher Peterson, Nansook Park, and Martin E. P. Seligman, "Orientations to Happiness and Life Satisfaction: The Full Life Versus the Empty Life," *Journal of Happiness Studies* 6 (2005): 25–41; and Christopher Peterson, *A Primer in Positive Psychology* (New York: Oxford University Press, 2006), 79, quoted in Shawn Achor, *The Happiness Advantage: How a Positive Brain Fuels Success in Work and Life* (New York: Random House, 2010), 40.
4. "Well-being," *Dictionary.com*, accessed December 20, 2021, www.dictionary.com/browse/wellbeing.
5. Sandra S. Maxedon, "A Study of the Gallows Transaction" (Master's thesis, Eastern Illinois University, 1978), 2, http://thekeep.eiu.edu/theses/3251. This thought-provoking master's thesis drives home the point that collusion with the gallows laugh reinforces self-destructive behavior and indicates that "performance levels improve when subjects become aware and stop using the gallows transaction." Mental health professionals who don't laugh along leave room for individuals "to smile at whatever is joyful rather than tragic" (p. 5).

Works Cited

Achor, Shawn. *The Happiness Advantage: How a Positive Brain Fuels Success in Work and Life*. New York: Random House, 2010.

Iyengar, Sheena S., and Mark R. Lepper. "When Choice Is Demotivating: Can One Desire Too Much of a Good Thing?" *Journal of Personality and Social Psychology* 79, no. 6 (2000): 995–1006. https://doi.org/10.1037/0022-3514.79.6.995.

Maxedon, Sandra S. "A Study of the Gallows Transaction." Master's thesis, Eastern Illinois University, 1978. http://thekeep.eiu.edu/theses/3251.

Recovering Couples Anonymous. *A Twelve Step Program for Couples*. 4th ed. Oakland, CA: World Service Organization for Recovering Couples Anonymous, 2011.

"Well-being." *Dictionary.com*. Accessed December 20, 2021. www.dictionary.com/browse/wellbeing.

9 The Recovery Cycle Illustrated

In This Chapter

- Vignette 1: Gerry, the People Pleaser, Learns to Say No
- Vignette 2: Sissy, the Entitled One, Begins to See Her Part
- Practical Decision-Making Can Be a Spiritual Event

A universe of choices opens with recovery. Knowing choices exist and determining the Price and Prize for any decision cultivates an ability to make decisions rationally (where we consider thoughts and feelings), not emotionally (where we react from fear). With this, recovering people come to realize this process is vital to living a more conscious, fulfilling, and love-filled life in recovery.

In the next two vignettes you will meet Gerry and Sissy. Their problems are very different, as are their temperaments. Both are in Twelve Step recovery and know about Prices and Prizes. Both have a sponsor (who is their sober guide in their program). Let's see how they problem solve as they grow in recovery and love. Using the Recovery Cycle as the backdrop, we'll pull it all together at the end and see how the entire cycle works.

Note: If you are not in a Twelve Step program, replace with another program of your choice.

Vignette 1: Gerry, the People Pleaser, Learns to Say No

Gerry is almost a year sober. He thinks about sobriety and the program a lot. He thinks about himself a lot too and spends a good amount of time identifying how he wants to be a man of his word. He attends meetings regularly where he learns about himself and how he relates to people.

Gerry has come to realize over the year that he has this habit of saying yes to things he doesn't want to do. He says yes to his parents, his friends, and everyone else when he really wants to say no. He tends to feel overcommitted and underappreciated; these feelings often compound into overtired, victimized, and resentful. Sadly, he often laughs when he uses the word *patsy* to describe himself.

A friend calls Gerry. The friend asks Gerry to take him to the airport tomorrow—during rush hour. Gerry knows that this will be a two-hour-plus chunk

DOI: 10.4324/9781003293231-12

of time—he did it a few times last month when he had a ton of other obliga-
tions. It was awful. Tomorrow, he has a day off planned. He's worked seven
days straight and has been savoring the idea of doing nothing. And now this!

I don't want to do it, I want my day off, he thinks. He didn't want to do it the
last few times but did it because he rationalizes, *That's what friends do.*

A Contrary Action for Gerry in this situation would be to say no. Or, a
sponsor might tell him it is okay to say, "I want to think about it and get back
to you."[1] These two responses are contrary or alternative to what Gerry would
normally do because he habitually says yes to everything.

The old behavior of saying yes to everyone may have been Gerry's reflexive
behavior while using and during that first year of sobriety. Maybe he believes
he can't say no because he was raised in a home that didn't permit him to say
no. Or perhaps he thinks people wouldn't like him if he said no. Or possibly
he has a dysfunctional belief about friendship, such as "Good friends always do
favors for each other." Whatever the reason, if he ends up feeling resentful ("I
want them to do it differently") or victimized ("Poor me"), Contrary Action
in some form is probably indicated. In this case, Gerry feels both resentful and
victimized.

He always does this. He should be asking someone else or taking an Uber, he
thinks. That is resentment.

Then he whines to himself, *Why does he always ask me?* That is being a
victim.

He suddenly realizes, *I'm a resentful victim.* Meanwhile, his friend is on the
line waiting for an answer.

Gerry Pulls It Together

In a flash, Gerry remembers what his sponsor told him after that last dreadful
trip to the airport. He remembers it is okay to say, "I want to think about it
and get back to you." Gerry somehow ekes out this strange sentence and tells
his friend he'll call him back in a few hours.

The friend says, "Okay."

It suddenly dawns on Gerry that he might have a choice!

He's heard his sponsor and others talk about all kinds of things he didn't
quite believe. Like the idea that there was a choice in the matter about almost
everything. This idea seemed too good to be true, like a pot of gold at the end
of the rainbow. But now he thinks maybe there is some gold in exercising his
choice.

But now what? He's committed to call the friend back. After a moment,
Gerry decides to call his sponsor to get some help.

Gerry's sponsor first congratulates him for exercising his choice to call the
friend back. Then he reminds Gerry there is a Price and Prize with every
decision. The sponsor asks Gerry to write out the choice (i.e., taking his
friend to the airport) and then identify the Prices and Prizes. Gerry puts it
this way:

Table 9.1 Choice: Saying yes to taking friend to the airport.

Price	Prize
I'll be resentful and tired	He'll like me
I won't get my full day off	I won't have to deal with the discomfort of saying no
I'll get stuck in rush hour traffic which I hate	People will think I'm a nice person
I'll get a stomachache[2]	

After sharing his writing with his sponsor, the sponsor asks who the "people" are on the Prizes list. Gerry doesn't know, but this gives him something to think about. Then the sponsor asks if Gerry believes the friend will only like him if he says yes to the request.

"Yes, that is what I believe," Gerry says.

His sponsor replies, "Hmmm, sounds like you really want him to like you. I have an idea. Why not sign up to be his full-time assistant—without pay. I'm sure he would really like you then."

Gerry and his sponsor laugh. The sponsor gives a little talk on people pleasing but Gerry just wants to know how to get out of feeling victimized NOW.

Then the sponsor says, "Okay, let's look at the Prices and Prizes for telling your friend no."

Now Gerry will be thinking the decision through from a different angle—from the perspective of saying no. (Remember, every decision has a Price and a Prize, and it is well worth it to flesh out difficult decisions.)

Gerry blurts out to his sponsor, "I'm taking up too much of your time. I feel ridiculous because this is such a silly problem!"

The sponsor replies, "I appreciate you want to take care of my time, however, I'm in charge of my own time. And you're in charge of yours—such as this situation with the airport. I want to work this through with you. And, I promise, this is useful and won't always be this long of a process. Call me back when you are done with your writing."

Gerry says, "Okay" and writes:

Table 9.2 Choice: Saying no to friend's request—no airport run.

Price	Prize
He may reject me; I'll lose him as a friend	I'll get my relaxing day off, which will feel good
People won't like me (Now, though, Gerry is wondering, *Who are the people anyway?*)	I'll be authentic—self-honesty
I'll feel anxious next time I see him	He may never ask me again—definitely a Prize
He'll think I'm a bad friend	I won't feel resentful and victimized!

Boom! After writing that last bit down about not feeling resentful and victimized, Gerry realizes his decision is made.

Any feeling, Gerry thinks, *is better than feeling resentful and victimized! Resentful and victimized gets me sick every time. I am willing to feel anxious and blaze into the unknown and do what is right for me. I am going to say no.*

Gerry calls his sponsor to report back and is reminded it isn't necessary to defend his "no," or to explain his reasons or feelings. The sponsor says, "No, it is inconvenient," is enough.

The sponsor says Gerry can, if he wants, soften it and say, "It isn't going to work for me."

Gerry decides to write down both responses so he can remember exactly what to say.

Gerry makes the call and uses the softer approach. The friend tries to get him to change his mind, but Gerry looks at what he has written and says, "No, it is inconvenient," without explaining. The friend backs off, Gerry wishes him a nice trip, and ends the call.

Whew! Done! Gerry is surprised at how relieved he feels. He decides, *I'm not going to call myself a patsy anymore.* Then he wonders, *Is this what self-esteem feels like?*

Pain, Pleasure, and All Feelings In Between

The sober person, like Gerry, may decide to take Contrary Action because *he is willing to have a different experience* at the other side of taking that Contrary Action. After taking the Contrary Action, we usually experience new and different feelings. Ideally, we learn to pause and identify those feelings. We also begin to learn that:

**How we think, and the decisions we make, are very much
related to how we feel about ourselves, the world, and others.**

Further, we learn to experience both pain and pleasure as part of life. We understand that all feelings come and go, don't kill, and are certainly never an excuse to drink, use, or act out.

Relief and Other Feelings

Pleased with how he handled the situation, Gerry begins to get very excited about his day off tomorrow. Then he thinks about the risk he took and how he thinks his friend will treat him in the future. He notices the good feeling slipping away. He feels anxious, uncomfortable . . . or is this dread?

But then he thinks about sleeping in and going to the beach tomorrow and about his sponsor's support too. He notices he feels good again, but then, doesn't quite trust it. He realizes his feelings are all over the place. Okay and then not okay. *But this is better than feeling an ongoing sickening resentment*, he thinks.

Overall, though, Gerry feels good about himself for making a choice in favor of himself, even with the discomfort. He wants to hold onto this positive thought and the good feeling it generates within.

Gerry senses sobriety will get easier with practice. He begins to acknowledge this entire experience as one of the Prizes of sobriety, even if it has been nerve-wracking. Gerry's thoughts continue to turn to more good thoughts about recovery, the program, his sponsor, and growing in self-esteem. Also, with a rush of gratitude he thinks, *Maybe there is a Higher Power on my side after all.*

The Recovery Cycle Backdrop—Transformation in Action

Now let's apply Gerry's vignette to the Recovery Cycle.

We started with Gerry thinking about his sobriety—his Recovery Focus. Then he was *triggered* to engage in people-pleasing behavior which in the past caused him to feel physically ill, emotionally upset, resentful, and victimized.[3] From information previously gathered at one of his Recovery Rituals (meetings), he realized he had been acting like a resentful victim. He then turned to another ritual—calling the sponsor. He weighed the Prices and Prizes from all angles. Contrary Action was indicated and suggested. He took Contrary Action and began to have a Range of Feelings, some painful, some pleasurable.[4] He could see the experience as valuable, even though sometimes uncomfortable. He appreciated he did it all sober. His appreciation multiplied into more good thoughts about sobriety and the program, which translated into some good feelings. Once again, he had a Recovery Focus when thinking about recovery, his sponsor, the program, and growing in self-esteem.

So that's how Gerry lives his simple recovery plan. This is how he will transform himself so he can stay sober, love better, and live the life he wants. A life not dominated by the "shoulds" of others.

Recovery is for sure simple, but not so easy when feelings come up, particularly mixed feelings. Recovery in this way, however, is always much easier than getting using/acting out or playing the victim for a lifetime.

Gerry's Backstory

What you don't know about Gerry is that he grew up in a home where he was given a lot of positive strokes for giving up what he wanted to do. He basically took care of his alcoholic mother and enabling dad. Also, he saw his dad structure a lot of time around doing favors for other people in the neighborhood, sometimes to the detriment of Gerry's family. Dad got a lot of strokes from neighbors, too. The less Gerry wanted or asked for, the more Gerry would be praised publicly and privately for being a good boy. Gerry's model of manhood was his father. Gerry's father, by example, taught Gerry to deny his feelings and wants in favor of everyone else's.

With the painstaking act of saying no to his friend, Gerry began to vote in favor of his feelings and wants. The cost for the new behavior was that he felt a little anxious, but he also felt good. He gained an emerging ability to be self-defined, rather than other-defined. In other words, he made a decision from the inside out, not from the outside in. This experience will lay the groundwork for Gerry's confidence in his own personhood and manhood in sobriety. If Gerry keeps making inside-out decisions for himself, he most likely will structure his time in a self-affirming, positive way. This will continue to build his self-esteem.

Also, the positive strokes provided by his sponsor were in many ways a corrective experience for Gerry. Gerry was rewarded for making his own decisions and doing the right thing for himself. Sponsors, therapists, and counselors can unseat adverse powers from the addict's earlier years. **Good guides help recovering people come to rely on their own decision-making capability**.

Gerry's experience is that of the more people-pleasing type of addict. The people-pleasing game is one of "If I do what you want, you will love me." People pleasers do this at a very high cost—they become self-sacrificial slaves, earning strokes by doing favors and manipulation.

Gerry's experience is obviously just one example of how the Recovery Cycle in tandem with a recovery program (in this case, Twelve Step) can work. But there's more.

The Entitled One

Not all addicts are of the self-sacrificial type. Some customarily think only of themselves—the furthest thing from their minds is considering the feelings of another unless there is something to gain. For this type, the best thing for growth might be to say yes to something where a no would be the norm. Hence, a "Yes, I will take you to the airport" or some sort of service to another would be Contrary Action for some. This emphasizes there is no right answer to any request, only what is right for us as individuals.

So then, what about this more entitled type of addict? Typically, this is a more rebellious, self-righteous one—although not always this overt. He approaches everyone and everything from a very different mindset than the people pleaser. This one believes: "It is their fault; they should be different. I'm right, I'm smarter, and people should serve me."

As the entitled ones barrel their way through life and relationships, they typically don't think they are part of the problem, but that's okay. Soon enough (or not), a loss of a job, relationship, or something meaningful may wake them up to their so-dry-ity. Yes, there's that word again. If you recall, one can be physically sober but dry. The good news is that the Recovery Cycle and idea of Prices and Prizes can work for this dry type, too, if there is even the slightest sliver of an open mind and modicum of willingness.

Vignette 2: Sissy, the Entitled One, Begins to See Her Part

Sissy has been clean and sober from alcohol for nine months. She thinks a lot about sobriety and how much more time she has on her hands now that she is sober. She also thinks she knows what could make the program better. She sees her sponsor weekly and has a home group. Now that she has committed to sobriety ("This time for good," she says), Sissy expects a daily parade filled with applause. She thinks everyone—especially her family—should forgive and forget and get over themselves. She is certainly no sissy—she blatantly corrects everyone, offers unsolicited advice liberally, and tells people what to do and how to do it. In short, Sissy is controlling.

Sissy created a lot of wreckage with her family while drinking. Sissy's daughter witnessed Sissy drive drunk and pass out many times. Her daughter, now an adult, just had a baby.

Now, Sissy wants to babysit her grandchild every weekend. Her daughter doesn't feel comfortable with Sissy babysitting at all yet—especially unsupervised and for overnights—and has said no. Sissy can't understand why and complains to her sponsor.

"She's being unreasonable. I'm the grandmother!"

Then Sissy adds, "I'll just show up at her house this weekend and insist! I know she'll see I'm right about this. I'll make sure her husband isn't there. I'm sure he is a big part of the reason I can't babysit."

The sponsor says, "Whoa! Before blaming your son-in-law, let's take a look at the Prices and Prizes of your choice to show up and insist your daughter does it your way."

Sissy reluctantly agrees to look at the Prices and Prizes. She wants to tell the sponsor that the Prices and Prizes exercise is not in the *Big Book of Alcoholics Anonymous* but decides not to correct her sponsor out of respect, for now. Sissy quickly states what she thinks are the Prices and Prizes. Then she can't help herself and blurts, "Prices and Prizes aren't in the Big Book, just so you know."

The sponsor smiles and says, "Thank you for pointing that out, Sissy. Do you want to know what I think the highest Price is?"

The sponsor had to point out the highest possible Price for Sissy to see it: That Sissy's daughter may cut Sissy off from a relationship with her granddaughter indefinitely. Because of Sissy's position of entitlement, she couldn't see the highest possible Price before. It dawned on her, after her sponsor pointed it out, that her daughter had threatened to do this the week before because of Sissy's meddling.

The sponsor also gave feedback about the Prize of NOT impulsively forcing the daughter to do it Sissy's way.

"If you respect your daughter's and husband's boundaries, there will be space for you to build a trustworthy relationship with your daughter and her family, and maybe one day you will be able to babysit."

"Okay," conceded Sissy, "I guess you are right. I'll do Contrary Action and do it their way. But I still think I'm right in that a grandmother should have certain rights, especially since I am sober."

The sponsor then told Sissy, "It's time you start your step work in the next few weeks so we can begin to work with the problem. And if you don't do the work, you'll have to find a new sponsor. It's your choice."

Sissy felt angry at her sponsor with this conversation. And although still fuming about her daughter's wishes, she did, however, make the choice to respect her daughter's boundary and start her step work. Not because of the sponsor's price tag, Sissy rationalized, but because she wanted to show her sponsor that she knew how to do the program.

Over the next several months, Sissy began to feel a bit uncomfortable because of the wreckage she had created with her daughter. She also began to see a lot of things, like that not getting her way was an emotional trigger for her anger. She began to have different feelings, too. Without trying to manage and control outcomes, she realized she felt anxious and sometimes sad.

Sissy continued to follow her daughter's lead about the visits and (as suggested by someone in her recovery group) graciously said, "Thank you" after each visit. She managed to accept and appreciate the time she got with her granddaughter, rather than trying to get her own way. She noticed that her daughter's husband was "actually a good guy."

With the new realizations, Sissy felt more appreciative of sobriety, the program, and her sponsor. She began to open herself up to the idea of a Power greater than herself, which she had openly resisted, and even began writing to this Power once a week.

We saw how Gerry's experience applied to the Recovery Cycle, but what about Sissy? If you were to apply Sissy's process to the Recovery Cycle, how would you describe it?

Practical Decision-Making Can Be a Spiritual Event

Gerry's and Sissy's experience show how the Recovery Cycle is steeped in the pragmatic. Their decisions were based on natural consequences and what would work for them in a real-world, heart-centered sense. Prices and Prizes don't allow for a make-believe world where what we wish for will always come true. We cut the best deals we can in life. Recovery is not about fantasy.

The cycle—with Prices and Prizes—allows for sensible, realistic, practical living. You get to figure out what works pragmatically for YOU. You get to consider your feelings and what will work for you in the details and bigger picture of your life. This can take time. For sure this manner of living requires some effort and thoughtfulness. At times you may feel like you are wrestling with unknown muddy monsters, and in a sense you are. Old belief systems and fear often will want to take over your mind and body. That's when faith can kick in and ease your struggle. We make the best decisions we can and make peace with not being in charge of the results. This recovery process is a down-to-earth, yet spiritual way to live.

The Spiritual Is in the Pragmatic

Whoa, you might be thinking, *Why are we all of a sudden talking spiritual?* Before you do any more thinking, hear me out.

Using the Recovery Cycle roadmap and having a program for living means getting to look within to decide what we want. We get to decide how best we can love ourselves and each other in the process of getting what we want. This can be a delicate balance, especially because the results we want are often not guaranteed. **Considering the loving and right thing to do—and doing it without a guaranteed result—is a big part of acting spiritually.** To do this is truly a miracle when considering how impulsive and self-destructive addicts can be.

Some of you may think this idea of getting what we want is selfish, but doesn't so much in our lives boil down to:

How much am I giving and how much am I getting?

Or:

How much am I loving myself and how much am I loving others?

Or, for those of you who know the immense value of serving others:

How do I love myself first and serve others, too?

It is practical—and spiritual—to weigh the cost for any decision in the way this book outlines. It just is. The process involves care and consideration of self and others. There's more to spirituality than this, however.

There is another Unseen Force of Spirit and Source of Power we can tap into for any decision. This Force is also available anytime when we want to control results. You can read the next chapter to gather more food for thought on the topic of spirituality. The good news about the spiritual stuff is there is no need to do anything you don't want to do.

The point is, if you want to live more spiritually, or even if you don't, consider doing the pragmatic by weighing Prices and Prizes. Love yourself enough to take the time to go within. Carefully consider yourself and others. Get support. Access help from something greater than your own limited thinking, especially if you are ruminating. Make a positive decision. Do something, or refrain from doing something (which can also be a positive decision). If you don't like how it unfolds, learn from it and move on. Recovery is simple when we stick to this plan. This is how we can transform from an addicted, fragmented mess into our original sense of wholeness, wonder, and love.

Recovery Recap

- Gerry gets support, considers Prices and Prizes, and learns how to say no. He honors his feelings, feels a new freedom, and grows in self-worth.
- Sissy relinquishes control, takes sponsor guidance, and does Contrary Action. She notices positive changes as a result.
- Spiritual living is in the pragmatic—we cut the best deals we can in life by weighing Prices and Prizes.
- In considering both the spiritual and practical ideas as outlined in this book, you now have a simple plan for recovery and living a spiritual life.
- If you don't want a spiritual life, that's okay—you still have a simple, practical plan in the Recovery Cycle.

Clinician's Corner

Boundary setting and graciously accepting the boundaries of others is almost an art and a big part of differentiating, individuating, and actualizing in recovery. In the clinical setting, we have an opportunity to model healthy boundaries. We do this within the client-centered space we create.

For Number 2, use a whiteboard or oversized wall Post-It and have clients describe their own Recovery Cycle process.

As usual, write out your answers for all questions before you give the questions to your clients.

Your Recovery Cycle (30–60 Minutes)

Write out your answers.

1. Give examples from your own experience about how you identify with Gerry or Sissy.
2. Describe how you are growing in the Recovery Cycle. Give an example in your life for each cornerstone. Include examples for triggers/cravings. Also, describe your experience of accessing help from someone.
3. What are your thoughts about the spiritual being in the pragmatic? Use an example from your life to describe.

4. What do you think about the question, "How do I love myself first and serve others too?" Do you have an example of this in your life in sobriety? If not, ask someone how they love themselves and are of service to other people.

Straight Shot (3–5 Minutes)

1. Draw the Recovery Cycle on a piece of paper. Write one example for each cornerstone as it applies to your life.

Notes

1. The sponsor's suggestion in this case is a wonderful strategy to desensitize to the idea of saying no. It buys time to work up to a no or to think about the request. We don't have to make decisions on the spot just because someone makes a request. We can benefit from taking the time we need to sort out how we feel.
2. Gabor Maté, *When the Body Says No: Exploring the Stress—Disease Connection* (New York: Wiley, 2003). Maté explores the negative effects on the body when people don't say no to psychological demands, rigid role definitions, and instincts gone awry. Basically, if we don't pay attention to our inner no, the body may suffer.
3. Triggers are not just about using—they can seduce addicts into behaving in all kinds of emotionally reactive ways (such as blaming, people-pleasing, intimidating, etc.). Addicts can pull the trigger, or they can choose to not pull the trigger. In other words, recovering people themselves are responsible for knowing their own triggers and managing them.
4. Often, newly sober people identify feelings as good/bad or comfortable/uncomfortable. It may take time to identify and name varied feelings, as well as come to know that many different feelings can be experienced at once. Mixed feelings are part of the human condition. If you have a difficult time identifying your feelings, Google a "feelings wheel."

Work Cited

Maté, Gabor. *When the Body Says No: Exploring the Stress—Disease Connection*. New York: Wiley, 2003.

Part Three
Spirituality

10 Not Your Ordinary Heaven

In This Chapter

- What Is Spirituality?
- The Spiritual Triad
- Faux Spirituality
- Wonders of Spiritual Living

Spirituality is a huge topic. We hear the word everywhere it seems. On Oprah, in self-help books, meditation apps, Russell Brand on YouTube, and most definitely in Twelve Step programs. What do you think when you hear this word? Does the word mean anything positive to you? Or do you think it is a fashionable word to primarily sell books or celebrity status? I've seen people roll their eyes at the mere mention of the word, as if it is a buzzword to ward off. For others, spirituality is about a profound, whole-souled, connected existence. For others still, the word evokes a kind of heavenly, cloudlike scene.

Recovering addicts do well with a positive view of the spiritual while incorporating it into their recovery plan. Acknowledging addiction as multifaceted—which includes the physical, mental, and emotional as well as the spiritual—will help in fulfilling a solid recovery with meaning. With an open mind and some willingness, incorporating the spiritual can be fairly easy.

Keep in mind that if you are in a Twelve Step program and don't like the Higher Power focus, there are meetings for agnostics. This means you neither believe nor disbelieve and may question the existence and nature of such a Power. Or, if you connect the idea of God and Twelve Step ideas with religiosity, which turns you off, consider how the Big Book of Alcoholics Anonymous was crafted in a more inclusive way, as to not exclude the sufferer.[1]

However, before any of you naysayers throw the book at me, give this chapter a chance. See what I mean by spirituality with its broad yet very personal definition. **Keep in mind that whatever your view, this chapter is not about convincing you of anything regarding spirituality**. Ultimately, spirituality is within the realm of your experience and what you make of it.

DOI: 10.4324/9781003293231-14

What Is Spirituality?

If we look at any definition of spirituality, we find it is a broad concept with many perspectives. Many sources agree that spirituality has to do with

- the human spirit or soul,
- finding meaning,
- something not explained by science,
- connection with something greater than oneself, and
- a universal experience.

One definition I like comes from a literature review (covering the effect of spiritual interventions on substance abuse recovery). The authors define spirituality as the "universal and fundamental human quality of searching for meaning, well-being, and profundity through connections with oneself, others, and the universe."[2]

Note: Spirituality is not religion, which is an organized institution with a system of beliefs. Spirituality, however, can be an element of religion, but one can live a spiritual life without identifying with or belonging to a religion.

If you consider yourself a neophyte about the spiritual, looking within and just thinking about spirituality and what it means may be a good first venture into matters of the heart, spirit, and something greater than you are alone. You may want to check out different definitions on your own and see just how many people out there are defining spirituality. I'm going to throw my two cents in, but I certainly won't be defining spirituality in its entirety. This would be impossible. Words seem insufficient to express its essence and complexity. I am no authority, but I do have my own experience.

For me, spirituality exists amidst mystery, miracle, and man. Like love, spirituality is a very personal yet universal experience. So much in recovery seems to be about paradox,[3] like the idea of heaven on earth.

Heaven on Earth

In active addiction, there is only personal hell, devilish limitation, and a wounded heart lost to an unforgiving world. In recovery, a heaven of infinite expansion and love can be found. In this place, all hearts can be healed, above ground, right here on earth. For addicts who have experienced this extraordinary transformation from addiction to recovery, it is certainly awe inspiring. It is, some might even say, the work of the divine—the stuff of a good and wondrous God. This mystical place and catalyst for such a metamorphosis in recovery is part of what I think of as spirituality. But there is more to this not-so-ordinary, earthly heaven.

Awe

Spirituality seems to be something beyond intellectual reasoning and partially about feeling and sensing. I hear people use the word *awe* with a feeling of connection to something outside or beyond themselves. I like the word *awe* a lot. Awe, and this unique connection, seem to be a part of spirituality for many in recovery.

If you have ever felt blissfully awed out and connected to everything in a good way, you may have had a spiritual experience. Unfortunately, the transient nature of the spiritual experience means it will come and go. So, as much as I like to feel awe (and maybe you too), my understanding of spirituality doesn't mean we are in a continuous, awed out, blissfully connected state.

The awe—as I experience it as a recovering person—comes from the realization that I am fundamentally okay and that I—that we—are not alone in our experiences, feelings, and especially in our suffering. This experience of wonder and "okayness" comes from feeling and thinking we are profoundly connected to each other—and to everything. We are a wave in slow motion in a big ocean.

Important note: Being fundamentally okay may not be an ever-present state of feeling fundamentally okay.

Being Okay Versus Feeling Okay

There is a difference between *being* fundamentally okay and *feeling* fundamentally okay. We can sometimes get this mixed up.

If we don't feel okay, we might think something is wrong with us and that our very being is not okay. Have you ever converted how you feel into a statement about who you think you are?

For instance, with some people, having feelings that don't feel okay (shame, for example) can get translated into thoughts like "I'm a mistake" or "There must be something wrong with me." This misguided, impaired thinking reinforces a self-destructive mode that can grind away at self-esteem and could lead back to using. Remember:

You can be okay even if you don't feel okay.

Many addicts come to know that connection (and the exchanging of life stories) with other recovering people somehow normalizes their state of being, however shame ridden or vulnerable they may feel. While identifying with another addict's sadness, frustration, joy, or any other feeling, there is often a feeling of connection. This connection is characterized by relief and a profound sense of "I'm not alone." This identification feels good. With this, awe can unexpectedly sneak up on a recovering person. For sure, though, awe comes and goes, just as all feelings do. Awe seems to play the game of peekaboo.

This peekaboo experience for many is magical, yet real at the same time. It often comes with the awareness that this special linkage (with another) is both lifesaving and awe inspiring. Over time in recovery, this awe can be compounded and can grow exponentially. Maintaining this connection and openness to a sense of wonder, however, can be a challenge.

When we don't feel awe after sharing our feelings, problems, and solutions with each other, we might think we are back to being alone (the fun peekaboo adult disappeared for good) and that somehow we were deceived. It might feel like the wellspring that absorbed all of our woes dried up, and we are left parched and alone in cactus land. The swapping of stories works sometimes, and helps us feel better sometimes, but the talking takes us only so far in the realm of the Spirit.

A Greater Source

This invisible wellspring of spirit connection (the exchanging of stories part) is only part of the bigger Spirit that animates us. We all can be connected to an even greater Source if we are open to it or willing to be open-minded about it. This Source of Power is greater than any individual alone, seems to have some say in the outcome of things, and at times, too, inspires awe. In a way, this Power is a shared current that connects addicts and all of humanity together and is available at all times.

Basically, there is something beyond the exchange and aggregate of human spirit that is included in this Power. Nature could also be included as part of this larger, shared current, as well as the entire universe of things we can't see.

This Unseen Force of power is part of the great mystery of spirituality:

> **There is me, there is you, and there is an invisible energy source that unites us all in a good way when we relate in love with each other.**

This current—this Power or Spirit—is what some in the Twelve Step program call a Higher Power. Others may use different names, like Mother Nature or Spirit of the Universe. Some recovering people call it God. For others who don't like the concept or word God because of a religious connotation or any other reason, they can designate a recovery group, or anything else, as the Power greater than themselves. Bottom line though: This Power is not you, or any one person. Maybe for you, it is science.

Faith

The maintenance of this connection—this relationship—to a Higher Power takes some effort. Faith in this Unseen Force will grow with time put into cultivating this relationship.

An Unseen Force

Your Power Source, should you choose to tap into it, can be almost anything you want it to be. What it is named, what it is, and almost everything about it is a personal choice. This means it can be a religious God or not. The only condition about this Source of Power is that it be greater than one's own self. That means as one human being, I have limited thinking, limited knowledge, and yes, limited power, and that another Force greater than me has access to much more information than my little brain alone.

Moreover, this Power is something I may not be able to comprehend because it is so much greater than me in so many ways. Accessing this Power takes the pressure off of having to figure everything out alone.

Think about how many times you tried to solve your addiction problem with your own thinking, all by yourself. Could you solve it? As Albert Einstein said, "We can't solve the problem with the brain that created the problem."

Accessing help from others or an Unseen Force might help with any problem you might have.

To get sober, we had to get help from other people's brains. For example, let's say this book is your first foray into recovery. The information in this book comes from years of data from a lot of other people's brains. The Recovery Cycle was inspired by information I've gleaned from the work of other people and their thinking and from witnessing others get and stay sober. This book and all of its unseen contributors—all those other brains—are collectively a Power greater than you. I'm not proposing you consider this book your Higher Power, but I am suggesting a new way to think about what your Higher Power could be. Again:

You get to choose your own concept of a Higher Power.
What it is, how it works in your life, and how you relate
to it is all your choice.

If accessing help outside of your own thinking has benefited your recovery in any way, chances are that same Power can assist with any other problem you might have going forward in recovery. This Power is not just in other people—you have another Source available to you as well. If you want to access this Source—however you define it—it is essential to develop a relationship with it. Many books are out there about how you can do this.

While developing this relationship, you may notice you are becoming increasingly okay with the unknown and unfolding. This is called faith. It is also possible you might notice your thinking and decision-making becomes more rational and sensible—in a word, pragmatic—because you have included this Power greater than yourself and have taken the time to love yourself enough, weigh Prices and Prizes, get help, make a decision, and then give over the results to a Higher Power. This is how faith can work.

Loving Ourselves, Loving Others

I am of the belief that when we love ourselves first, we can love others better. Figuring out how to love ourselves and others can be perplexing for any recovering person. Sobering up is one sign of self-love. It is your first step into your heaven. And enlisting the help of something greater than ourselves can be advantageous as we explore new ways of living, loving, and relating in recovery. As we explore this unbodied dimension, though, we must also step toward others.

Back to Earth

Spirituality is not just about me loving myself, feeling awe, and believing there is something greater than me. A big part of spirituality in recovery includes others. Unless we've chosen to be a monk in the mountains, we will run into others at work, doing errands, taking the kids to school, talking to a roommate about the dirty dishes in the sink, and the like. We bump into other spirits of humankind all of the time.

Part of being spiritual in my book—and this is my book—is not only about caring about ourselves but also about caring about each other and treating each other honestly and kindly. **This is one great essence of spirituality: caring about ourselves, caring about each other, and demonstrating that.** Sounds doable, right?

Some of you might be thinking: *But what about when he says he'll be home at 6 PM and gets home at 7:30 PM? Or when I'm on hold with the phone company for an hour and then I get cut off? Or when she disrespects me? Or when he dumped me by text? We all can't be little angels in these kinds of situations or in the heat of a maddening argument!*

I get it. We live on earth with other people who get in our blissful way. In recovery, however, we can learn to be honest and act kindly even in the most infuriating of situations. Learning how to do this just requires effort, practice, and a little faith. No matter how far away from awe we feel in any given moment, and even when emotions flare, it is possible to be honest and kind toward our fellows, even with that most bothersome institution or family member. And if you fall short of the ideal? Tools in your program can help you look at your part, clean it up, and get back on track.

There is a woman I know who frequently says, "Spiritual is as spiritual does, follow me home." This means we can talk all we want of spiritual matters at meetings or even from a book, but watch me in my daily interactions with others, especially at home. According to this woman, and I agree, how we treat others, especially the ones we are most comfortable with and when no one is watching, is a benchmark of our spirituality.

Spirituality exists in right action.

The spiritual way is doing the right thing at home and everywhere in our lives. Our actions, here on earth, are what define us.

The Spiritual Triad

Some of what we've learned so far in this chapter is that spirituality in recovery includes this threesome:

- a Higher Power (or whatever you want to call a Power Source greater than you),
- self, and
- others.

You have a choice to embrace or reject the spiritual, but frankly, if you are in a recovery program with others who are sober, you might just catch yourself in a spiritual moment and begin to like it. It might feel good, maybe even a feeling you would call spiritual. Then you will want more of it. (As addicts, we always want more of what feels good.) Then, you might just find yourself doing more to get a spiritual feeling again.

The spiritual is what makes recovery easier than going it alone.

Where there once was reliance upon your finite self and thinking, there is now support from a Source of Power greater than you can imagine, with good feelings to boot.

Let's take a glance at the three parts of this all-inclusive, ethereal system that I believe are necessary for a simple and easy recovery: A Higher Power, self, and others.

A Higher Power

Again, name your Power Source whatever you want as long as it is greater than you. This is your personal choice.

If we are to cultivate a connection with this Higher Power, we might want to have an idea about the nature of this Power. This is another great thing about identifying your own Power Source: You decide what characterizes this Power. I heard a woman say once, "Pick a God that loves you." I like this a lot. Some people come to recovery with a punishing or ignoring God. This is not helpful. Can you imagine why it might be easier to establish and maintain a relationship with something loving rather than punitive or remote? My thought is, come up with a Power that is at the very least neutral or objective. Loving words that evoke a feeling of being supported might be better though. If you have any trouble with this, ask someone in recovery about their Higher Power or their faith.

It may at times seem like there is too much emphasis on spirituality. For those of you who might eye roll or eyebrow raise at this Higher Power focus, you might want to reconsider. Musings about spiritual matters are not a waste of time but an investment in a richer, more meaningful recovery. I can tell you this all day, but again, this is something you will come to experience for yourself with some investment in time.

Self

Much of recovery rests on getting to know the self, caring for it, and allowing that self to shine in the sun. Deep within each of us, all genuine wants reside. This is where one's unique personhood dwells, one's original sense of wholeness. The creative and highest self is there. This oft-buried self is, paradoxically, the most brilliant side of our selves.

Think of yourself as a geode. A geode is a rock on the outside with beautiful concealed crystals on the inside. These hidden facets of YOU are inside you. Inside you is the gem. Most likely, it will take time and some personal work to expose this lighter, crystalized self so it can freely reflect itself to the world and, yes, shine brightly in the sun.

One of the easiest ways to start this rediscovery and reclamation of the self (that gem in you) is to work the steps in a Twelve Step program. This is done with a sponsor or spiritual guide and your Higher Power.

Throughout the work, with whatever program you choose, there will be some quiet time. This alone time is for introspection and developing a relationship with oneself and the Higher Power of your choosing. With all the mobile devices and other distractions of today, how could anyone get to know one's self, much less a Higher Power, without some downtime in reflection? This contemplation time is part of becoming intimate with ourselves and our spiritual Source.

Others

Getting to honestly know one's self, and sharing that self with the world, is a big part of recovery. The irony is that we get to know ourselves with alone time, but we need relationships with others to get to know ourselves. We need others in recovery, and others also need us.

Addicts often consider people quite bothersome. I know I have. One man in a rehab group I was leading said, "My problem is people." The entire group roared with laughter and identification. Many of us would agree it is a lot easier to be spiritual alone. But not many decide to go off into the hills and live a reclusive lifestyle. The rest of us deal with families, friends, co-workers, other drivers on the roadways, and people blocking the aisle with a shopping cart at the grocery store. In emotional times, we want these people to get out of our way and behave according to our wishes. But to deal with (what we think are) annoying people—or rather, to relate to them in a caring way—is part of spirituality in recovery.

How do we learn how to share this planet with others and find awe in our day-at-a-time sobriety? As addicts in recovery, we learn how to do this with others who are in recovery. We need these others, so it is probably a good idea to learn how to get along with them. In recovery, we find others who have our same problems but who have come up with solutions. Through them, we discover solutions for ourselves, and then pass on what we've learned. We become of service to others. With these others, we hear laughter. By just being with recovering people, we learn to have fun where there once was none.

Faux Spirituality

For any of you who might still stiffen when you hear words like spirituality and serenity, you might have good reason. Human beings aren't perfect models of spirituality (and serenity) at all times. Maybe you think there is some kind of fakery at play, or perhaps you don't like the words and what they mean. Whatever your reason, I think I might understand. After all, we are finite, fallible, flawed human beings, not perfect people.

Talking the Walk Is Not Walking the Walk

If you are on board so far, then you get that being spiritual doesn't necessarily mean sitting high on a mountain top all alone chanting "Om," although it could be. And it certainly isn't spouting spiritual principles and truths without walking the walk. Here's a real story that speaks to this point.

A man was having this beautiful share about his Higher Power. The timer beeped, signaling him to stop his share. He continued sharing—it seemed no end was in sight—and the leader politely let him know his time was up, for the second time. This rational man with a terrific message suddenly morphed into a vicious werewolf and snarled at the leader, "I'd like to rip your head off." Everyone recoiled and shuffled uncomfortably. I think a few members even looked for the exit but realized leaving would put them within the man wolf's sightline, which I'm sure they thought would make matters worse. Everyone waited for the monster's next growl, but he just sat there, huffing something inaudible to himself. In a flash, the leader continued to call on other people, as if the vile display hadn't happened. The primitive animal, now turning back into a man, backed off. The puff of his grisly chest shrank with each passing moment, and the meeting resumed without further incident.

When the stench of an over-inflated ego reeks, we may acknowledge the stink, but it's always good to remember that a dose of patience and compassion help clear the air. (I know I haven't always been the most fragrant gardenia in the room. What about you?) Be kind to others and yourself when the odorous ego flares in all its atrocious glory. A foul ego just means a deep wound. Like some recovering people say, "We don't shoot our wounded," even if they appear weird and werewolf-like.

This does not mean hanging out with toxic people. If you are scared, it's important to walk away. Don't try to save them or go to battle with these people unless you want to be bloodied in some way.

In recovery, we walk the walk as best as we can. We are all human animals, not flowers in sweet bloom 100% of the time.

Beware the Spiritual Bypass

Some sober addicts talk about spirituality in a way that sounds more like denial and fantasy. Spouting spiritual truisms can be a way to escape reality. This may work in the short term, but it does not substitute for nor is it the lifeblood of human spiritual experience. Eventually pretense wears thin. This avoidance of true feelings and real spirituality by quoting spiritual-isms is what one of my clients called a "spiritual bypass." It is this kind of pretending and denying of one's inner humanity, through a spiritual veneer, that circumvents and stunts authentic spiritual growth. We all struggle and have wounds. It is okay to be human and not have all of the answers. No one does.

Honesty

Learning how to be honest in all areas of one's life and over one's lifetime is fundamental to spiritual progress. Remember that idea of a person impersonat-ing a person? When you are not being true to yourself, it can grind away at a deep place within. It requires a tremendous amount of inner work, courage, and faith to be honest with oneself and others.

Once we get honest with ourselves, communicating honestly with others becomes the next big challenge. Being honest with others, without dis-counting ourselves or others, will propel us into a spiritual (albeit human) realm of existence. **Creating the space to be honest with oneself, others, and one's Unseen Source will be a huge part of the addict's spiritual solution.**

Wonders of Spiritual Living

With our minds and hearts aimed toward living a spiritual life—a life where we practice acting in a kind, honest, compassionate, and fair-minded way toward self and others—all while bringing a Higher Power into the loop—we notice many wonderful things. We experience a greater capacity to bear and accept a wider Range of Feelings. Suffering has more meaning and the joys are that much sweeter. Strength is found in vulnerability. We are more congruent with what we value and hold dear.

In living spiritually, we are pleasantly surprised to have a deeper connection with ourselves and others. We like this connection. Creativity can flow. Authenticity, spontaneity, and being true to oneself are more the norm rather than vague memories of a distant childhood. Mistakes are opportunities for growth and grace. Impulse control is fairly easy and inspires a balanced existence. An increasing confidence in the process of life and recovery has taken hold, and goals of perfection have been discarded. Under these conditions, we can finally relax so positive love can flourish. Does this sound like some otherworldly, extraordinary heaven?

Keep in mind, though, living spiritually is not a perfect place or something anyone can do perfectly.[4] Perfect spirituality is not the goal. The idea is to keep seeking and experience what spirituality means to YOU.

I'm hopeful this chapter sheds light on the spiritual solution in recovery. On this note, let's move on to the next part of our journey, which is all about love and intimacy.

Recovery Recap

- Spirituality is a broad concept with many perspectives.
- Spirituality is beyond intellectual reasoning and partially about feeling or sensing a connection to something greater than oneself.
- How we demonstrate caring about ourselves and each other is one great essence of spirituality.
- The spiritual makes recovery easier than going it alone.
- Spirituality exists in right action.
- The Spiritual Triad includes a Higher Power, self, and others.
- One easy way to reclaim the gem that is YOU is to work the Twelve Steps in a recovery program with a sponsor or spiritual guide or participate in some sober-focused group with others.
- Aiming our minds and hearts toward living a spiritual life means we practice acting in an honest, compassionate, and fair-minded way toward self and others, all while bringing a Higher Power into the loop.
- There is no perfect spirituality—spirituality is an ongoing process of seeking and expansion to be experienced by YOU.

Clinician's Corner

Increased utilization of spiritual resources and rituals has been shown to have positive outcomes for recovering people.[5] For those who don't believe addiction has the spiritual malady component, spiritual rituals enhance well-being in general and make for a more emotionally stable existence,[6] so why not consider it as just another tool to feel better? In other words, keep it pragmatic.

For some clients, it might be best, however, to stay out of whether or not addiction is a spiritual problem. Keep in the center, though, a proposed difference between the mind and the brain:

The mind can be considered a "relational and embodied process that regulates the flow of energy and information,"[7] whereas the brain is an actual physical structure in the body.

With this, our brains, capable of jumpstarting behavior with thought, could be understood as the mechanism which guides us, independent of anything or anyone else. In other words, one might consider the matter of sobering up a manifestation of ones own thinking (i.e., their own psychological process, generated from their brain) whereas another might consider it a spiritual event (i.e., some unexplainable energy flow struck them sober).

Explore with your client their ideas about spirituality. Suggest spiritual sources and encourage spiritual practice (or a psychological approach if your client rebuffs the spiritual).

Discuss the difference between mind and brain with your client, as stated earlier.

As usual, you answer the questions first. Remember to not let your personal views seep out of you and into your client's process.

Spiritual Action (15–45 Minutes)

Write out your answers.

1. What does spirituality mean to you? What is your experience of it?
2. What do you think about the idea that spirituality exists in right action? Describe what this means to you.
3. How do you incorporate the spiritual into your recovery and life? Do you have a belief in a Higher Power? What is your name for this Power?
4. Choose one spiritual practice such as silent/guided/walking meditation or a spiritual reading and do it either alone or in session with your therapist. After, discuss the experience.
5. Reach out to someone in recovery and ask how they are, or, volunteer to be of service in some way to your recovery group.

Straight Shot (3–5 Minutes)

1. Discuss your thoughts about spirituality and the idea of a Higher Power with your therapist or sober guide. Do you think having a Power Source greater than you can be helpful? How? Pick one current situation and share how a spiritual approach might help.

Notes

1 William H. Schaberg, *Writing the Big Book: The Creation of A.A.* (Las Vegas: Central Recovery Press, 2019), 152–153. A must read for anyone wanting a scholarly, detailed, blow-by-blow account of the development of the Big Book and the spiritual flavor of the Twelve Step program.
2 "Weighing the Evidence for Spiritual and Religious Interventions for Substance Use Problems," Recovery Research Institute, accessed December 20, 2021, www.recoveryanswers.org/research-post/spiritual-religious-substance-use-outcomes/.
3 Alcoholics Anonymous World Services, *Experience, Strength and Hope: Stories From the First Three Editions of Alcoholics Anonymous* (New York: Alcoholics Anonymous World Services, 2003), 155–156. "We must die to live, suffer to get well, surrender to win, and give it away to keep it." These paradoxes recovering people know so well are described in the story, "The Professor and the Paradox." This book is a compilation of stories from the first three editions of Alcoholics Anonymous.
4 Ernest Kurtz and Katherine Ketcham, *The Spirituality of Imperfection: Storytelling and the Search for Meaning* (New York: Bantam, 2002). A much deeper discussion on this topic of spirituality, imperfection, and recovery can be found in this book. This is a beautifully realized work for any imperfect perfectionist who wants nutrient-rich spiritual food for thought and comfort.
5 John F. Kelly, Robert L. Stout, Molly Magill, J. Scott Tonigan, and Maria E. Pagano, "Spirituality in Recovery: A Lagged Mediational Analysis of Alcoholics Anonymous' Principal Theoretical Mechanism of Behavior Change," *Alcoholism: Clinical and Experimental Research* 35, no. 3 (2011): 454–463, https://doi.org/10.1111/j.1530-0277.2010.01362.x; Elizabeth A. R. Robinson, Amy R. Krentzman, Jon R. Webb, and Kirk J. Brower, "Six-Month Changes in Spirituality and Religiousness in Alcoholics Predict Drinking Outcomes at Nine Months," *Journal of Studies on Alcohol and Drugs* 72, no. 4 (2011): 660–668, https://doi.org/10.15288/jsad.2011.72.660.

6   Agnieszka Bożek, Paweł F. Nowak, and Mateusz Blukacz, "The Relationship Between Spirituality, Health-Related Behavior, and Psychological Well-Being," *Frontiers in Psychology* 11 (2020): 1997, https://doi.org/10.3389/fpsyg.2020.01997. I love this study! Why? Because its findings "carry important implications for the faculty members responsible for curriculum preparation to account for teaching contents related to the conduct of a healthy lifestyle and to spiritual development." Translation: It might be a good idea to encourage discussion of spirituality into substance abuse/addiction studies in the classroom.
7   Daniel J. Siegel, *Mindsight: The New Science of Personal Transformation* (New York: Random House, 2010), 52. This definition adds a whole new dimension to the word "mindful."

Works Cited

Alcoholics Anonymous World Services. *Experience, Strength and Hope: Stories From the First Three Editions of Alcoholics Anonymous.* New York: Alcoholics Anonymous World Services, 2003.

Bożek, Agnieszka, Paweł F. Nowak, and Mateusz Blukacz. "The Relationship Between Spirituality, Health-Related Behavior, and Psychological Well-Being." *Frontiers in Psychology* 11 (2020): 1997. https://doi.org/10.3389/fpsyg.2020.01997.

Kelly, John F., Robert L. Stout, Molly Magill, J. Scott Tonigan, and Maria E. Pagano. "Spirituality in Recovery: A Lagged Mediational Analysis of Alcoholics Anonymous' Principal Theoretical Mechanism of Behavior Change." *Alcoholism: Clinical and Experimental Research* 35, no. 3 (2011): 454–463. https://doi.org/10.1111/j.1530-0277.2010.01362.x.

Kurtz, Ernest, and Katherine Ketcham. *The Spirituality of Imperfection: Storytelling and the Search for Meaning.* New York: Bantam, 2002.

Recovery Research Institute. "Weighing the Evidence for Spiritual and Religious Interventions for Substance Use Problems." Accessed December 20, 2021. www.recoveryanswers.org/research-post/spiritual-religious-substance-use-outcomes/.

Robinson, Elizabeth A. R., Amy R. Krentzman, Jon R. Webb, and Kirk J. Brower. "Six-Month Changes in Spirituality and Religiousness in Alcoholics Predict Drinking Outcomes at Nine Months." *Journal of Studies on Alcohol and Drugs* 72, no. 4 (2011): 660–668. https://doi.org/10.15288/jsad.2011.72.660.

Schaberg, William H. *Writing the Big Book: The Creation of A.A.* Las Vegas: Central Recovery Press, 2019.

Siegel, Daniel J. *Mindsight: The New Science of Personal Transformation.* New York: Random House, 2010.

11 Love, Intimacy, and Sexuality

In This Chapter

- What Do Love and Intimacy Have to Do With Recovery?
- What Is Love?
- What Is Intimacy?
- Four Requirements for an Intimate Relationship
- Twelve Questions for Intimate Relating
- What About Sexuality?

Love, intimacy, and sexuality can be elusive elixirs for many addicts, even well into recovery. They can be confusing and exasperating. If we want positive, loving relationships in recovery and healthy sexuality, too, then learning about and practicing the art of loving is a good idea. With some humility here, I will attempt to partially unravel the shroud of mystery around these big topics.

What Do Love and Intimacy Have to Do With Recovery?

If you want something beyond dry abstinence, you might deduce that love and intimacy have everything to do with recovery.

We used our drug of choice often because we hated ourselves, our partners, the checkout clerk, and whoever else agitated us. With no love of ourselves or humankind, how could we stay sober? The distress that comes from a lack of love can be too much to bear because it can turn into self-destructive hate without us even knowing it. This hate can trigger us to use. Moreover, without learning to love in a positive way, it is impossible to foster emotional sobriety. This lack of emotional sobriety means we end up nurturing and settling for limited, volatile, or stagnant relating. This kind of connecting might even seem normal.

As for intimacy, when using or dry, we weren't intimate with ourselves or others. We didn't know how to be. Intimacy requires honesty and vulnerability (and we know how that can go for addicts). When we are not rigorously honest, we lie about our addictions, our relationships, and a lot more. When we

DOI: 10.4324/9781003293231-15

can't be vulnerable, we aren't teachable, and therefore cut ourselves off from learning how to be intimate. Without a willingness to take emotional risks, we can't really know ourselves and therefore can't be intimate with others. Keep in mind:

Without learning how to love and be intimate with yourself and others, you may use again or stay a dry drunk.

Do you know why this might be? If you remember from Chapter 3, cultivating healthy relationships plays a big part in any meaningful recovery. In our addictions, we avoided people and being real with ourselves and others. This unhealthy way of relating clearly didn't work, or you wouldn't have ended up addicted, desperate, lonely, and now reading this book.

If you choose to continue on that same lonely roundabout, you will keep getting the same result—doing life alone, going round and round, resentful at others you see on roads more interesting and fun, blaming them for having cars better than yours. In other words, you will be terminally dry or on your way to Addiction Street again.

Taking the time to learn how to be in healthy, loving, and intimate relationships means turning on to Recovery Road with your Recovery Cycle. This route is the way to living freely and joyously with yourself and others. It will be essential in helping you recover and discover more of who YOU are so you can live the life YOU want.

At this turning point, there is only one question: Do you want to take that right turn and ease onto the road toward better loving, intimacy, and sexuality? You are the driver.

Funhouse Relationships

It might be fun going into the warped mirrored funhouse at the circus, but I don't think any of us would want to stay there for very long because we might get sick. How addicts go about getting love and intimacy can be a bit wacky, but not always in a fun way. Yet addicts—sober or not—will stay in the weirdly mirrored relationships that don't feel good and make them ill.

Have you ever felt so churned about a relationship that your torso felt like an empty, gaping hole with a frosty wind blowing through it? Or did you ever overeat because of an argument, to the point of throwing up? Or maybe your heart hurt when you realized your dream boat was really an old, rusty, half-sunken ship, stuck in shallow waters—try as you might to stay fixated on the little bit of bow above the waterline, you couldn't ignore the behemoth that was clearly dead in the water. Or, does fantastic chemistry dupe you time and time again into thinking *This is the one*, when, upon a closer look after the glow, you see someone so incompatible or emotionally unstable you can't believe you've fallen for the chemical con one more time?

Any of the aforementioned experiences could happen in an hour, in a week, or over a lifetime, maybe even with the same partner. Desperate to feel love, we want to see what we want to see. But if we are still in the funhouse full of distortions, everything is going to look deformed, no matter where we fix our gaze.

We all want the experience of love, addict or not. And many of us think we want intimacy, but don't really know what that word means or what it entails. So . . .

Without the skills on how to be in loving relationships, we often build what we think is love on a distorted or broken foundation.

Fear is typically at the core of why we do this. The results are that some addicts anxiously long for the fantasy partner or relationship, while others create distance and remain avoidant to stay in control. I'll address these two types in a minute. For now, though, know that these two ways of relating can look and feel resentful, bitter, coldly quiet, hostile, or highly dramatic in some other way. I don't think many of us would consciously choose these styles of relating, but somehow recovering people end up doing just that. But there is a better way.

Building a lifetime of love and intimacy on a solid foundation is possible.

Having a realistic understanding of what love and intimacy mean will help you move toward them in a positive, concrete way. This is the beginning of stepping out of the slanted funhouse.

What Is Love?

This is a big question, right? Have you ever tried to define love? Have you ever looked it up? When you think about any definition of love, or how you love, or who you love, does the definition fit? How about when you are in disagreement with who you love? Does your definition work then? Is love to you a feeling? An action? A commitment? An art? Is love something you can make happen? How many different types of love do you think there are?

The Bible says there are four types of love. Google says there are six, eight, or twelve. Those in the mental health profession have come up with their own ideas about love. For example, Erich Fromm, author of *The Art of Loving* (which you may want to read), describes the theory and practice of love in nuanced detail. Some spiritual teachers do a fine job of imparting wisdom from the ages about how we can love better. There is a ton of information out there about love. Addicts, not always but often, have a murky or skewed sense of what love is (any sex and love addicts identify?), particularly in romantic relationships. This twisted sense of love, spun in the subconscious mind, can trump all good information.

A Warped Sense of Love

For anyone who has listened to any recovering people, it is probably no surprise to hear that a warped sense of love can stem from childhood wounds. With many addicted people, inadequate reflection by remote, absent, or uber-controlling parents (or caretakers) may have been the norm. Or, perhaps inappropriate touch of a violent or sexual nature powered the home's contaminated emotional staple. Or, maybe the child was completely ignored, which can be the cruelest, most loveless desert of all. Skewed ideas of love seem to come from these kinds of fragmented foundations.

Note: This is not to blame the parents for the addiction, but simply to point out that children who are not positively and sufficiently reflected or touched might have a distorted sense of love, and how to love, as adults. Many addicted people seem to have found their drug or acting out as a solution to deal with the pain of not experiencing a positive brand of love in childhood.

Pain = Love

Many addicted people seem to learn early on to equate pain with love.

As human beings, babies need sufficient emotional reflection to feel secure in relationships.[1] We need to be seen. We also need adequate physical touch to live and thrive.[2] Ideally, this reflection and touch is affirming. Good reflection and touch are a vital mix for healthy attachment and hence positive loving.

Love in a dysfunctional home, as suggested earlier, equals pain in a *felt* sense. What is *felt* from the parent's behavior—shame, anxiety, or fear, let's say—is paired with some idea of love (e.g., "Mommy hits me but says she loves me so therefore this painful experience is love"). The internalized message becomes: *The way I feel, the way she acts and the way I have to act to feel secure (i.e., to get the "love" I need) is how to be in a loving relationship.*

This equation for love (i.e., pain = love) is then carried into adult relationships. Sadly, these adult relationships are often characterized by DIPS (the Drama, Intensity, Pain, Struggle from Chapter 7) and for some, addiction/compulsive behavior. Children who grow up in a discounting/dysfunctional family system as described earlier can grow into adulthood having difficulty creating healthy bonds in relationships, especially in romantic relationships.

Attachment and Upgrading Relationships

Warning: This is for anyone who wants a basic understanding of attachment theory and those wondering why they might be struggling in romantic relationships.

Attachment theory describes three fundamental attachment styles: avoidant, anxious, and secure.

- *Avoidant:* "I am nervous when people get too close and people fail me, so why bother."

- *Anxious:* "I often worry that people don't really love me. I believe if I am who they want me to be, they will love me."
- *Secure:* "I find it relatively easy to get close to others and am comfortable depending on them and having them depend on me. I don't worry about being abandoned or about someone getting close to me."[3]

You might have guessed by now that our early attachments with our caregivers have everything to do with the way we relate—and love—in all of our relationships, but more specifically, in our romantic relations (whether prone to addiction or not).

If you used your addiction in any way as a solution to knock out your pain (and/or intrusive thoughts) from any childhood wounds, you most likely fall into the avoidant or anxious category. Or, you may identify with both of these. The good news is that you have upgraded from complete denial to now becoming aware. So now, if your drug is relatively a nonissue, you can learn about your attachment style and do something about your pain (and how you think about it). Let's flesh out the styles of avoidant and anxious a little more.

The avoidant one runs away from pain and may avoid relationships, have a string of short-term stands, or remain in a long-term relationship while maintaining a good amount of distance.

The anxious one longs for the perfect relationship, whether in a relationship or not, usually hoping the idealized mate will someday want him/her/them as badly as he wants him/her/them. This anxious one leans into the pain of longing; in a twisted way, the deficit felt equals love.

And so goes the addictive cocktail: The avoidant pulls away, while the anxious longingly designs the chase to capture the love. Needless to say, the avoidant and anxious are perfectly yoked. The problem, though, is both feel unhappy and trapped but accept this painful, codependent experience as love.

Can you think of any time you might have been a part of the mix in the avoidant/anxious lovemaking drink? Do you want to drink a different drink?

Before, while using your drug, you may have had a wonderfully addiction-riddled relationship drink. Now sober, you may have a garden-variety codependent relationship brew. This concoction, though, is better because now you are conscious. With this new awareness, you now have an opportunity to create the healthy green drink you want. There is a way to feel secure in love.

**In recovery, we can learn how to love better and
feel more secure.[4]**

These early experiences live in the subconscious mind and seem to drive how we relate in love. Breaking the subconscious patterns of our minds and actions, especially for recovering people, takes time. This is part of learning something new. And little by little—over time—it's how we learn in recovery. We desensitize to positive love experiences. Remember? Think baby steps, or little sips of wheatgrass.

> **Love is an experiential journey to be discovered and owned by YOU.**

Learning How to Love

Being in relationship, and applying what we learn along the way, is how we learn to love. Having a vision of where we want to go and a good map will make it easier for us to take steps to get there.

What if you wanted to go on your dream vacation? Let's say it is Tahiti. Wouldn't you want to know what airline to take to get there and where best to stay? If you know you are prone to bug bites, wouldn't you want to bring some bug repellent? And what about clothes? You would probably guess that a swimsuit and shorts would be better than snow gear.

Because you know what a sunny Tahiti is like, even though you haven't been there, you have a general idea of what to expect and how to prepare yourself. You also know that there may be some rain and will equip yourself with rain gear. You did the research.

It's the same thing with love. We have an idea of what we would like, but the reality of love is that depending on our emotional weather at the time, we might experience rain or rainbows. It just takes time throughout our sober journey to learn how to best travel toward our ideal love destination.

Let's face it—sometimes that perfect destination seems unreal. It's a process to go from fantasy to reality, but that's what learning to love in sobriety is all about. With support, and yes, with learning more about who you are with Twelve Step or other help, love lives become less about disappointing venues and more about all-inclusive resort loving.

Bottom line: This work is deeply personal. It's not easy, but it's worth it. Recovery really is the ticket to Happily Ever After. (Not that Happily Ever After exists in the way you might think. Enter intimacy.)

What Is Intimacy?

Let's start this topic with one thing intimacy is NOT.

> **Intimacy is NOT round-the-clock googly eyes and gushy feelings that last continuously and indefinitely.**

Nor is intimacy just good sex. Good sex can be part of an intimate romantic relationship, of course, but it is not a full-bodied definition of intimacy.

Addicts can get mixed up thinking romance and good sex are what intimacy is all about. This kind of thinking is fantasy, and addicts love the high of fantasy.

Let's Get Real

Many books and articles have been written about intimacy. A range of definitions exist, so I'm throwing in one I like. From what I know, **intimacy boils down to clear, caring, honest communication about what we want and don't want**. In other words, a willingness and practice of honestly communicating who we are. This is both pragmatic and spiritual. With this, the essence of intimacy plays out in this practical, heart-centered way:

> Person 1: "This is what I want and this is what I don't want. What do you want, and what do you not want?"

> Person 2: "This is what I want and this is what I don't want. What do you want, and what do you not want?"

Both: "Let's make a deal."[5]

Wants and Not Wants[6]

A "want" is something the kid—that authentic self in YOU—wants. You may want one thing, and everyone else may want something different. You have a right to what you want. This concept, though true, is hard for many addicts who may have been discounted as kids to grasp. Your wants are what make you YOU.

"I want" doesn't always mean "I get," however. This is where negotiation and compromise come in.

A "not want" is the thing you don't want. This is when a small voice inside signals "no," or the idea or thing doesn't feel good in your body. It's a good idea to pay attention to "No, I don't want . . ."

Listen to your inner no, for it holds the golden key to your integrity and self-esteem.

Holding a boundary based on "no" is good for overall well-being. Remember, though, negotiating is all about compromise. This could look like, "I say no to this, but I can say yes to that."

When it comes to negotiating wants and not wants, keep an open mind. Sabotaging relationships based on insisting on getting our way might not result in getting what we want in the bigger picture. At the same time, sacrificing ourselves and our integrity by agreeing to something that is a clear no probably won't result in us getting what we want either, unless what we want is a resentment.

A great thing about recovery is you are in a position to check in with your own heart, brain, and Higher Power so you can negotiate for what you want and don't want.

A Note on Wants Versus Needs

Some of you may be thinking, *What about my needs?* Or, *What is the difference between expressing my wants and my needs?* The answer is multilayered, and a bigger discussion than I want to get into here, but consider these tidbits.

1. There is a tendency to throw around the word need as if it was a life-or-death matter. For example, "I need a manicure!" or "I need sex every day" or "I need you to . . ." (which is never a good one for a relationship). These are wants, not needs. Needs are in the category of what we need to survive, like oxygen or water.
2. Also, it can be a slippery slope into a wall of resistance anytime we say, "I need you to . . ." (or for that matter, "I want you to . . ."). How do you feel when someone says, "I need you to shape up"? That is not a need but telling someone to be more, better, or different.
3. For an intimate relationship, for sure there are some requirements/elements needed. The Four Requirements for an Intimate Relationship are described at the end of this chapter.
4. If you want more on wants and needs, google Maslow's Hierarchy of Needs or "wants vs. needs."

The point about this is to get you thinking about language. With all of this, you get to:

> **Ask for what you want and say no to what you don't want when negotiating.**

"Let's Make a Deal"

The "let's make a deal" part includes both people sharing thoughts and authentic feelings about the topic and then coming up with a feel-good compromise agreement for both parties. This requires that we know what we want and don't want before any deal-making can take place. This way of negotiating is a rational yet feeling-centered process.

Some addicted people have difficulty even knowing what they want and don't want, however. Spending some quiet time in reflection may help to sort this out. Getting to a point where we can directly and cleanly negotiate is nothing short of miraculous, considering some early programming.

It might be that an addict's wants and not wants were discounted in early life. For example, a mom says to the little girl who wants red shoes, "You don't want the red shoes, the blue shoes are better." With this, the little girl feels bad and starts to cry. Mom then says, "Oh, you shouldn't be upset, honey, you can see that blue really is the better color."

Can you see how this little girl could grow into not trusting her own yes and no about what she wants and doesn't want, in shoe color and in life?

This kind of discounting of personhood can result in children growing into adults who truly don't know what they want or don't want (or they may know their wants/not wants but find ways to hide them from others.) This is not their fault, though. They had trainers. The challenge for these addicts is to find out what they want and don't want for themselves (or, for the hiders, to openly reveal what they want and don't want). This is a big deal for them. An even bigger deal is learning how to negotiate authentically, directly, and lovingly with others.

Without knowing one's wants and not wants and negotiating cleanly for them, intimacy can't exist. Codependence in the form of martyrdom, passive aggression, extreme narcissism, or any number of distancing tactics and roles can breathe and thrive, but not intimacy. The general tenor of relationships based on a lack of clean negotiation can be silent, seething, and resentful or highly dramatic and overtly emotional.

Our wants and not wants, along with thoughts and feelings, are what make us individuals. We make choices that determine the course of our lives based on our wants and not wants. These choices come from honoring our thoughts and feelings. The addict who has been cheated out of this experience of being oneself—of embracing and inhabiting one's very spirit—can be tragically out of touch with himself and others.

Addicts seem to go one of two ways with this discounting program: submissive or rebellious. The stances seem to be determined by temperament and environment.

Are You Submissive or Rebellious, or a Little of Both?

The more submissive type aborts the process of looking inside by fulfilling everyone else's wants. This is the placating people pleaser. This one seems to know what everyone else feels and wants and is at the ready to help others, to the detriment of selfhood. Often it takes time in sobriety for the submissive type to get in touch with their own feelings and wants and then to authentically express them. This one is prone to self-sacrifice. Think Gerry from Chapter 9.

The rebellious sort, on the other hand, presents as if they know exactly what they want. They often resort to bullying tactics and negotiating with an intimidating, "It's my way or the highway" intensity. This can be overt (bully-like intimidation) or covert (passive aggression). Negotiating is a challenge because of a firm belief in the stance, "My way is right." They may think they are being taken advantage of or controlled in some way if they give in. For this one, the challenge may be letting go of control, taking small risks by considering the other side, and having an open mind so creative solutions can surface. This one leans toward self-sabotage. Think Sissy from Chapter 9.

A little of both—This person swings back and forth between submissive and rebellious.

Do you identify? If yes, how?

So now that we know there is a difference between intimacy and fantasy, we can now look at one very important aspect of intimacy—vulnerability.

Vulnerability

Vulnerability, in psychological terms, means being open to attack or harm emotionally. Do you know any addict, or anyone really, who wants to open themselves up to attack or harm? This sounds threatening, doesn't it? Opening ourselves up to attack or harm could mean death—as if our very being could be extinguished or swallowed up.

This may sound absurdly theatrical, but this is what is happening in the subconscious mind of an addict when deep fears are running the show: *If I reveal my most tender insides to you, you will take advantage and gut me.*

From depths below the surface, fear often energizes the most terrified part of ourselves that works to keep us safe from attack, more wounds, and death. Many of us used because we were afraid of something and didn't feel safe. We didn't want to feel vulnerable. In recovery, though, and in life: **It is okay to feel vulnerable.** As Brené Brown said, "Vulnerability is at the core, the heart, the center, of meaningful human experiences."[7]

Fear and Addiction

If we think of fear being at the core of addiction, then we can look at an addiction's motive in a different way.

If we turned to our addictions because we were afraid of something, we could actually think of our using as trying to keep us safe from whatever made us afraid. Perhaps the addiction wasn't really out to harm us but wanted to keep us feeling safe and comfortable. What worked and felt good in the beginning, though, got out of hand.

Although the circumstances of your life may have changed for the worse because of your addiction, the addiction's motive remained constant: "I don't want you to be afraid. I am here to comfort you."

From this viewpoint, we might see the addiction was just trying to be helpful—and for a while it was. But in the end, it almost squished all the life out of you.

The more afraid we become, the tighter the addiction's grip.

Remember Lennie in John Steinbeck's *Of Mice and Men?* He loved petting soft animals, but he would accidentally kill them. He didn't know his own strength. He was just being Lennie. Like Lennie's strength, addiction's powerful grip can squeeze you to death, even though it means to caress you gently.

Regardless of what you are afraid of and how tightly addiction has you in its grip, it's important to remember that you are not your addiction. You are YOU. It is up to you to take responsibility for moving toward the love and safety that helps you heal and grow.

In recovery we identify our fears and learn how to keep ourselves safe.

But What Are We Really Afraid of?

By working the steps in a Twelve Step program, therapy, or another recovery program, an opportunity exists to identify fears specific to our personal situations.[8] We realize we have all kinds of fears. We are afraid people won't like us. We are afraid we won't get the perfect spouse, pet, or seat at the movie theater. We are afraid we made a wrong decision and will be forever regretful. We are afraid people will laugh at us. We are afraid we will get the job or won't get the job. We are afraid of getting old and ending up in a nursing home. The list of fears is endless.

Two main, deeper fears relating to vulnerability and intimacy are the fear of being abandoned and the fear of being engulfed. These two fears can be so entrenched in the subconscious mind of an addict that vulnerability is almost impossible without being honest with oneself and getting help from others. Depending on the level of discounting, temperament, and help sought, it could take years to fully grasp how these fears (and feelings of not feeling safe) are connected to patterns of communication in adult relationships.

Are You Afraid of Being Abandoned or Engulfed?

These fears of abandonment and engulfment mean you believe you will die if Mommy or Daddy leaves you; or, you will die if Mommy or Daddy consumes you. Abandonment equals death. Engulfment equals death.

You might have a deep fear of being abandoned if you were at any time afraid of Mommy and Daddy abandoning you (or they did abandon you). It makes perfect sense that you would do anything to please Mommy and Daddy so they stick around. Your very life depends on keeping Mommy and Daddy fed and happy.

You might have a deep fear of being engulfed if you felt that Mommy and Daddy could swallow you up, as if they were scary monsters keeping you prisoner, just waiting to devour you and your spirit. Tactical fighting with the goal to get away would be your plan. Your whole life depends upon avoiding the monster's foul, hungry growl.

With either fear of abandonment or engulfment, the motto in the subconscious grotto of the mind is: *If to be myself is to die, I will do whatever it takes to live.*

Do you identify with either a fear of abandonment or engulfment? Or both?

Now sober, have you ever thought someone important in your life (other than Mommy or Daddy) was going to abandon you or consume you? If yes, what did you do with your fear?

For us to be intimate with each other, we must learn to be ourselves so we can reveal ourselves, and vice versa. If we learned to be a version of a person or are constantly avoiding others, we aren't being or revealing ourselves. If we want intimacy—the ability to freely expose who we are and what we value—we will first want to reclaim ourselves in all our messy glory (and take a risk that we won't die in the process). For intimacy to occur, we must be vulnerable somewhere. That means experiencing some yucky feelings.

Reclamation

By now you know that the first part of reclaiming oneself is to abstain from using the drug. This is the beginning of waking up to oneself (and is a wonderful act of self-love, too).

The next big part of this reclamation process is opening up about your addiction with others. We let others in on the dirty little details of our using that only we know. The who, what, where, when, why, and how of it. And how we felt too. This honesty, which requires vulnerability, is required for getting closer to knowing what you want and don't want in life. This fundamental part of honesty in recovery will put you one step closer to intimate relating in all of your relationships.

Coming clean about the addiction with another somehow helps addicts feel good enough to reveal all kinds of secrets and thoughts held dear. We risk that people won't leave us or eat us up when they know what we've done, what we think, and who we are in all areas of our lives and relationships. Then, we somehow feel safe. **The recovery paradox here is, we must take an emotional risk (which feels scary) to feel safe and more secure in ourselves**.

Another part of the reclaiming is to become vulnerable with ourselves. This is about being in acceptance of ourselves as is. We don't have to fake that we know everything and are in control. Staying in control (as if we really have control) is a way to stay invulnerable. Sometimes falling apart is necessary for growing into who we want to be. And we learn that in falling apart we don't die.

How can a recovering person who is unwilling to explore the depths and heights of their own life experience be able to sit with and be open and intimate with another? If we haven't sat with ourselves and our stuff (perhaps because it is too painful), aren't we still hiding from the scary monsters, bound to repeat the dysfunctional patterns we learned long ago? And isn't staying within our own pattern another way of staying in control and alone? And for some, wasn't that aloneness—the hole inside you were trying to fill—part of the reason for the addiction?

We've been looking at intimacy and vulnerability in general, which could apply to any relationship, romantic or otherwise. For a bigger discussion on romantic relationships, though, it might be wise to understand in greater detail the idea mental health professionals know: We must be an "I" before we can be a truly intimate "we."[9] (Our partners in romance seem to be the ones who hook us into feeling the most emotionally off-key and blissfully in tune.) The Twelve Steps can be a big part of discovering how to be an I. As you become that I, just remember that your partner (and others) may not like it.

True, some partners may leave and not like who you are or what you want for yourself. You might find yourselves incompatible. This may happen, but you will be okay. It is important to know you won't die if the partner leaves. If your partner bails (or you at a nonemotional time find the incompatibility unbearable), the relationship wasn't meant to move forward. On the other hand, one may stay and work it out with you. You both might compromise. As you learn to make deals, you both might discover how to respect and cherish each other. Then, how would *that* feel?

Four Requirements for an Intimate Relationship

Intimate relationships require vulnerability, safe dialogue, reciprocity, and consistency.

Vulnerability: For the addict, the vulnerability piece is huge. This is part of the personal work. Without being grounded and in acceptance of deep feelings during a discussion with the other, fear will rear to get feelings under control. Ergo, getting the environment under control is next, and getting exactly what the addict wants will be the goal, rather than a meaningful discussion which could lead to an agreeable comprise or a creative outcome. Honest, productive negotiating is just not possible with defensive or offensive gloves in play.

Safe Dialogue: Safe dialogue is talking to one another in an honest, kind, even-minded way without intimidation or guilt-inducing tactics. Safe dialogue is not laying down the law, giving choices without discussion, going into a monologue, not speaking up about one's true feelings out of fear, or any other offensive or defensive maneuver. Learning how to effectively dialogue may take communication skills training, both verbal and nonverbal. This will take both personal and relational work . . . and practice, practice, practice.

Reciprocity: Reciprocity is when both in good faith can share thoughts and feelings to explore whatever is being discussed, including any fears, pain, anxiety, or any good stuff that comes up. This is a give-and-take process, ideally where both feel safe enough with each other to expose themselves, *and both do it*. This is not a one-sided process but a relationally intimate one that involves both partners sharing themselves. If vulnerability and reciprocity aren't happening in the dialogue, going to a couples therapist may be helpful. Without reciprocity, intimacy will be elusive at best.

Consistency: Consistency with safe dialogue and reciprocity inspires trust so vulnerability can occur. Consistency provides structure, reduces anxiety, and desensitizes us to healthy, rational communication experiences.

The point about this intimacy stuff is for addicts to have a clear idea about what intimacy is and how to do it. Once you know, then decide if intimacy is what you want. If it is, then you are now in a better position to practice being intimate.

Twelve Questions for Intimate Relating

If you are interested in an intimate relationship, it might be a good idea to ponder these questions:

1. Do I feel like I can be myself in this relationship?
2. Do I feel comfortable asking for what I want and saying no to what I don't want?
3. Do I like myself when I'm around this person?
4. Can I share my feelings with this person without feeling shamed or afraid?
5. Do I feel supported? Do I support the other person?
6. What kind of relationship do I want and am I willing to state this desire openly?
7. Am I willing to learn how to have conflict and work through disagreements?
8. Does this person have a trustworthy record? Do I?
9. Does this person make and keep agreements? Do I?
10. Does this person negotiate in a kind, feeling-centered, and rational way? Do I?
11. Are we compatible enough?
12. Are our values aligned enough?

If an intimate relationship is what you want, are you willing to take a risk on another human being? If so, then go for it with a conscious and active intention to do it over time. Be sure to bring vulnerability, safe dialogue, reciprocity, and consistency to the process.

Intimacy is not a perfect state or process, no matter how much information one has on the subject. Being in an intimate relationship doesn't mean defenses won't flare. If a defense sparks, it doesn't mean a couple, for example, isn't intimate or does not have the capacity for it. Growth toward more intimacy is possible if the recovering person has a sound vision of what intimacy is and is willing to do what is suggested. It's okay to not be perfect. No one is.

For couples, if one is interested in an intimate relationship and willing to work for it and the other is not, it's best to accept the relationship and person as is. Figure out how to live with it or reject the relationship. Expecting an intimacy avoider to change into your fantasy partner is a recipe for resentment and long-term pain.

That said, some couples have found intimacy and healing thanks to the Twelve Step program of Recovering Couples Anonymous. Intimacy avoiders beware: In this program, both must be willing to work together for their couple-ship to sail peacefully into the sunset.

What About Sexuality?

I don't know one addict who hasn't at one time or another had questions about, difficulty with, or a general discomfort around their sexuality. When I say *sexuality*, I mean your capacity for and management of your sexual feelings and behaviors. Many good books out there delve into this topic and are well worth checking out, especially if you are recovering from sexual compulsivity.[10] In this section, though, we'll look at how you can move toward healthy sexuality vis-à-vis the Recovery Cycle.

Whatever sexual difficulty you might have, the Recovery Cycle can help you move toward your ideal—as you experience the heal in the real.

Sex in sobriety can be a sticky subject. Who wants to honestly discuss their sex life or thoughts about sex? Even in the room with a therapist, shame can choke, preventing open talk of sexual matters. Sex talk with anyone can be hard.

I remember in graduate school when the professor asked us students to write down—and say out loud—all the dirty words we could think of. I basically froze—I could barely bring myself to form the syllables, much less say some of the words with confidence in front of my peers. They were all having at it, as if in some orgasmic situation. Me? I'm not a prude, but I didn't want any part of the party. I did it, though, and within a week was practicing all kinds of words around the house, all to my husband's surprise (and delight, I gathered). Now, anything having to do with sex and body parts I can hear and say with ease. For you therapists out there, this is very important!

In that situation, applying the Recovery Cycle, my focus was learning to be a therapist. I knew clinicians must be comfortable with any sex-related words or situations a client brings into the room. I was attending class, the ritual (i.e., consistent activity) required for a degree, which now was asking me to step out of my comfort zone. I took Contrary Action and said words—and said then some more. My feelings? Afraid and vulnerable at first, then strangely comfortable. Even though we were all clearly very different, I felt a greater connection to my fellows in class and to my newfound ability to say and hear sex-related words.

Healthy Sex

Before we understand how to apply the Recovery Cycle to sexuality, check out the healthy sex list in Table 11.1. This will help you move toward your feel-good ideal for sober sex.

If you think about your current or past sex life, could you say you hit all the marks on the aforementioned list? If not, and you want to be sexually active now in a healthy way, which items do you want to move toward?

Many aspects to sexual dysfunction, discomfort, and health come to play for recovering people. Psychological challenges can be roadblocks to healthy sexuality; in particular, faulty belief systems can not only perpetuate the Addiction Cycle for sex addicts but also sustain various degrees of discomfort/dissatisfaction for sober people in the bedroom. Moving toward the sex you want—that is good for you—may require help from a professional who specializes in sex, especially

Table 11.1 What is Healthy Sex? Reprinted with permission from Alexandra Katehakis,
        Inc. 2016.[11]

Is consensual	Empowers each partner
Is an individual choice	Includes healthy boundaries
Is equal and mutual	Is safe, but not too safe
Is respectful	Celebrates individuals and their bodies
Is responsible	Includes expressions of appreciation for self and partner(s)
Is intimate	Enhances each partner's true self
Is nurturing, healing	Reflects the values of each partner
Is trust-building	Is an expression of love and/or caring
Is not manipulative or exploitative	Includes good communication
Includes sharing	Has an ultimately controllable energy, even if it gets wild
Is authentic and honest	Does not produce feelings of toxic shame or guilt
Is not pathologically dissociative	Does not produce health issues
Is not trauma repetition	Respects gender identity and sexual orientation
Enhances self-esteem	Includes the giving and receiving of pleasure

if you've experienced sexual/childhood trauma, or if you experience problems related to sexual compulsivity, or both.

In the meantime, whether you choose to get help or not, you can apply the Recovery Cycle to your sexual problem.

Applying the Recovery Cycle

Starting with the "What is Healthy Sex?" list in Table 11.1, you can begin to envision the healthy sex life you want (Recovery Focus). Make a point to do something regularly to learn more about what healthy sex is for you (Recovery Rituals). Maybe this is reading the books at the endnote section of this chapter or accessing help from a sex therapist. Then, maybe you would ask your partner to engage in regular intimate time where you can express your sexual desires, in an honest, safe way.[12] Or, perhaps you want to abstain for a while as you set boundaries for yourself. As you know, with any Contrary Action, feelings will bubble. But, by this time, with your recovery tools and support, you will have a greater capacity to experience discomfort or pleasure or any feelings that come up for you (Range of Feelings). And because you have a growing ability to manage your feelings, you can get back to your mindful focus on the healthy sexuality you are beginning to experience. All of this is you experiencing the "heal in the real" around your sexuality and recovery.

Note: If sexual compulsivity has been a problem, it's best to reach out to your sponsor, sober guide, or a professional before embarking on any self-guided sexual recovery plan.

Sex, like any problem in recovery, requires we get honest with someone about what has been a problem, or what has been weighing on our hearts and causing stress. Honesty is part of the healing solution.

You are worthy, and it's okay to have a fulfilling sex life in sobriety if you want one. The question is, are you willing to feel what you need to heal to have it?

I hope the last few chapters have provided some guideposts on how to discover what love, intimacy, and healthy sexuality mean to you. For recovering people, having specific, healthy ideas and behaviors for love, intimacy, and sexuality may help in the ongoing process of realizing them in a concrete way.

Recovery Recap

- Part of recovery is learning how to love ourselves and each other better.
- Without learning to love and being intimate with yourself and others, you are bound to settle for limited, stagnant, or volatile relating. Worse, you may use again.
- Without skills on how to love, we build what we think is love on a faulty foundation.
- Having a realistic understanding of what love and intimacy mean will help you move toward them in a positive, concrete way.
- Three basic attachments styles are anxious, avoidant, and secure, and we can learn how to feel more secure and love better.
- Defining love, and learning how to love, will be your personal and experiential journey.
- Intimacy is not Fantasyland but often a pragmatic process where we openly reveal what we want and don't want and negotiate cleanly for it.
- The Recovery Cycle can help you move toward healthy relating and sexuality.
- The four requirements for an intimate relationship are: vulnerability, safe dialogue, reciprocity, and consistency.
- Intimacy is not a perfect state or process. Sometimes defenses flare. It is okay to be imperfect as you grow in love and intimate relating.
- The Recovery Cycle can help you nurture the positive love and sexuality you want, and there will be feeling in the healing.

Clinician's Corner

A growing ability to love self and others *in a positive way* may be at the heart of every client's recovery solution. Think of your experiences with love. Who helped you in becoming a more secure you, where you felt okay to be, feel, think, and share in your own way? By creating a safe space for clients so they can honestly share, feel, think, and finally *be*—their own way—you can assist them toward better loving, intimacy, and sexual health.

As usual, answer the subsequent questions for yourself before giving them to your clients. And, since this is the final Clinician's Corner, I have a few questions just for you:

How has it been giving up that thing you decided to give up at the beginning of this book? How has the Recovery Cycle helped? And what have you learned about yourself and how you love and are intimate? How do you feel about your sexuality?

Love Your Way (30–60 Minutes)

Write out your answers.

1. To love in a more positive way, the way you want, what would you be doing differently? This could be loving yourself better, or others. Do you think your understanding of love is realistic? Why or why not?
2. Review the attachment styles: anxious, avoidant, and secure. Describe your attachment style. Give examples.
3. Do you feel safe to reveal what you want and don't want in all of your relationships? If not, what prevents you from being honest? Is it a matter of knowing how to communicate your preferences and feelings in a straightforward, kind way? If yes, who could you ask to help you with learning how to express yourself?
4. Review "What is Healthy Sex?" in Table 11.1. If you think about your current or past sex life, could you say you hit all the marks on the list? If not, and you want to be sexually active now in a healthy way, which items do you want to move toward, and how do you want to do this?
5. Think about any important relationship you have (or have had). Is (or was) there vulnerability, safe dialogue, reciprocity, and consistency? Describe. If you don't (or didn't) have all four, what would you change in you so you could move toward intimacy? Is intimacy, as described with these four elements, something you really want?

Straight Shot (3–5 Minutes)

1. Choose one idea or page from this chapter and write about how you
    relate.

Notes

1   This statement is a basic tenet of what is known in psychological terms as "attach-
    ment theory." For more on the science of attachment theory as it relates to sex/
    love addiction, read Alexandra Katehakis, *Sex Addiction as Affect Dysregulation: A
    Neurobiologically Informed Holistic Treatment* (New York: Norton, 2016). In Chapter
    2 ("Basic Neurophysiology of Attachment and Affect Regulation"), you will find
    a beautifully crafted scientific explanation about how the bond between caregiver
    and child affects the brain and can set the stage for sex/love addiction. This book
    is aimed at a professional audience or those interested in scientific detail. Katehakis
    has other books on sex addiction and healthy sexuality that might be more acces-
    sible for the more casual or self-help reader.
2   Ashley Montagu, *Touching: The Human Significance of Skin*, 3rd ed. (New York:
    Harper & Row, 1986), 96–197. The entire chapter speaks to the idea of the human
    need for adequate physical touch for one's overall health and livelihood.
3   Mario Mikulincer and Phillip R. Shaver, *Attachment in Adulthood: Structure,
    Dynamics, and Change* (New York: Guilford Press, 2007), 27. A scholarly work on
    attachment style, this book describes the attachment styles of avoidant, anxious,
    and secure in glorious, comprehensive, study-rich detail. Most addicted people new
    to recovery don't seem to fall into the secure category.
4   Daniel J. Siegel, "Making Sense of Your Past," *PsychAlive*, accessed December 20,
    2021, www.psychalive.org/the-importance-of-making-sense-of-our-pasts-by-daniel-
    siegel-m-d/. To love in a positive way is something that can be learned, for sure.
    This positive learning curve can lead to an attachment narrative called "earned
    secure." Broadly speaking, "earned secure" emerges with making sense of how one's
    dysfunctional childhood plays out in the present, along with some emotional risk-
    taking (with trustworthy, secure individuals) in the here and now. Those who are
    anxious or avoidant can learn what it is to be secure, but it must be earned. This
    earning comes with emotional labor and time in recovery.
5   Pat Allen, in conversation with the author, circa 2008.

6   Pat Allen, *Conversational Rape: Emotional Language, Conditional Love and Invasive Communication Patterns* (Newport Beach, CA: The Dr. Pat Allen WANT® Institute, 2012). How we get what we want and don't want is all about how we communicate with others. If you want to learn the specifics about how to talk straight in a loving way (and not crooked in a game-playing way), read *Conversational Rape*. Part of the purpose of this gem of a book is "to identify and quantify those factors that cause pain and inhibit intimacy in human relationships" (p. 10).

7   Brené Brown, *Daring Greatly: How the Courage to Be Vulnerable Transforms the Way We Live, Love, Parent and Lead* (New York: Random House, 2015), 12. Brown researches vulnerability (courage, shame, and empathy) and has excellent questions centering around the topic of vulnerability (pp. 289–303), which I suggest you check out, if you dare.

8   In the Twelve Step program, Steps Four and Ten are inventory steps. In part, these steps ask recovering people to identify specific fears. In working all of the steps with a sponsor or spiritual guide, the subject of fear typically comes up in conversation. Sponsors and guides offer shared experiences and strategies to help the addict overcome their fears. Some acronyms for FEAR are: False Evidence Appearing Real, Feeling Excited And Ready, and Face Everything And Recover.

9   David Schnarch, *Passionate Marriage: Keeping Love and Intimacy Alive in Committed Relationships* (New York: Henry Holt, 1997), 53–74. Schnarch's stimulating read covers human sexuality, differentiation, and how to be an individual while in a romantic relationship. This idea of being an "I" before being a "we" is what recovering from codependency is all about and is echoed in many books and in therapists' offices as well.

10 Alexandra Katehakis, *Erotic Intelligence: Igniting Hot, Healthy Sex While in Recovery From Sex Addiction* (Deerfield Beach, FL: Health Communications, Inc., 2010). Patrick Carnes, *Out of the Shadows: Understanding Sexual Addiction*, 3rd ed. (Center City, MN: Hazelden, 2001). For those in recovery from sex addiction, these books offer deep insight and tools for sexual healing.

11 Alexandra Katehakis is the clinical director of the Center for Healthy Sex (located in Los Angeles, CA) where a team of dedicated professionals specializes in sex therapy and sex and love addiction treatment.

12 Tammy Nelson, *Getting the Sex You Want: Shed Inhibitions and Reach New Heights of Passion Together* (Beverly, MA: Quarto Group, 2008). "I" statements, validation and empathy prime the pump for more satisfying dialogue and sexual experiences á la Imago Relationship Therapy fashion. In addition, David Schnarch's *Resurrecting Sex: Solving Sexual Problems & Revolutionizing Your Relationship* (New York: HarperCollins, 2002) is another resource for just what the title says.

Works Cited

Allen, Pat. *Conversational Rape: Emotional Language, Conditional Love and Invasive Communication Patterns*. Newport Beach, CA: The Dr. Pat Allen WANT® Institute, 2012.

Brown, Brené. *Daring Greatly: How the Courage to Be Vulnerable Transforms the Way We Live, Love, Parent and Lead*. New York: Random House, 2015.

Carnes, Patrick. *Out of the Shadows: Understanding Sexual Addiction*. 3rd ed. Center City, MN: Hazelden, 2001.

Katehakis, Alexandra. *Erotic Intelligence: Igniting Hot, Healthy Sex While in Recovery From Sex Addiction*. Deerfield Beach, FL: Health Communications, Inc., 2010.

Katehakis, Alexandra. *Sex Addiction as Affect Dysregulation: A Neurobiologically Informed Holistic Treatment*. New York: Norton, 2016.

Mikulincer, Mario, and Phillip R. Shaver. *Attachment in Adulthood: Structure, Dynamics, and Change.* New York: Guilford Press, 2007.

Montagu, Ashley. *Touching: The Human Significance of Skin.* 3rd ed. New York: Harper & Row, 1986.

Nelson, Tammy. *Getting the Sex You Want: Shed Inhibitions and Reach New Heights of Passion Together.* Beverly, MA: Quarto Group, 2008.

Schnarch, David. *Passionate Marriage: Keeping Love and Intimacy Alive in Committed Relationships.* New York: Henry Holt, 1997.

Schnarch, David. *Resurrecting Sex: Solving Sexual Problems & Revolutionizing Your Relationship.* New York: HarperCollins, 2002.

Siegel, Daniel J. "Making Sense of Your Past." *PsychAlive.* Accessed December 20, 2021. www.psychalive.org/the-importance-of-making-sense-of-our-pasts-by-daniel-siegel-m-d/.

12 The Path From Here

The path from here is about what you will do with this information and what path you will choose in your sober journey, right now.

If you've made it this far, the Recovery Cycle makes some sense to you. Recovery has meaning for you personally and is precious. Therefore, you are okay with doing the deal of working for your recovery. This means you

- maintain a Focus,
- do Rituals because they are meaningful to you,
- weigh Prices and Prizes in making decisions,
- take Contrary Action,
- feel a deepening Connection (with yourself, others, and a Source of Power greater than you alone),
- have a willingness to feel a Range of Feelings, and do your best to accept all feelings as part of your human experience, and
- stay willing to maintain your Focus and grow more into a sober YOU.

Even on days that you don't feel particularly inspired or spiritual, you know that you will feel better eventually, and that it will "all come out in the wash," as my grandmother used to say. Your clean and sober plan is always there for you.

As we now know, the choices we make and the relationships and love we cultivate dictate the quality of our lives in recovery. In some cases, the choices we make could be the difference between life and death. Recovering people who have been close to death know this too well. Hopefully, those days are in the past for you. So, what about right here, right now?

Right Now

You are on your path, right here, right now. You have a choice in this moment and in every moment. Granted, you might not always like the choices, but you do have choices about everything, even in your most awful moments when there seems to be no choice.

Viktor Frankl, the Austrian psychiatrist and Holocaust survivor, made the choice to find meaning in existence under the most horrific situation imaginable. If you've read his book, *Man's Search for Meaning*, you may know that he

DOI: 10.4324/9781003293231-16

made a choice about finding meaning in the most dehumanizing and cruel place. His here was in a concentration camp. In the camp, he found love as a link to having a hold on one's spiritual self and, with hope, a will to live honorably.[1] These are just a few of the many takeaways from Frankl's brutal experience.

The point I want to make is that even in the midst of suffering—be it a family member's death, a seemingly loveless marriage, or anything else—there is always a choice in attitude and perspective (and what to do or not do). Even with situations less traumatic. Granted, most of us haven't had anything close to Frankl's unimaginable experience, but we can look to his awareness and insight as a spiritual and inspired message for any kind of suffering, duress, or emotional pain.

One day I injured a disc in my spine. I was mindlessly doing a yoga pose and pushing my body far beyond what it was capable of handling. I could barely walk for a few weeks after the initial injury, having to wait for the inflammation to subside before doing anything but the basics for homebound living. When I could finally get up enough to lay myself on the ground, a therapeutic yoga practitioner gave me something to do: Lie down on the ground on my back with knees bent and visualize alternating lifting one foot off the ground at a time. He wanted me to visualize but not actually move!

Here at that time was downright depressing. I fashioned myself athletic and thought I could overcome anything. But there I was, seriously incapacitated, hunched over in some old flannel pajamas, barely able to walk, visualizing. Valium (this dates me, I know) was really sounding good, but of course, it was not an option. I did what was suggested and eventually, after two years, could do moderate forward bends. This was a challenging time, and it was frequently difficult to make the choice of seeing the experience as an opportunity for spiritual growth and healing. I cared about myself enough to access help. At that time, "here" in every moment was an opportunity to change my perception—there was always a choice.

That experience taught me much about yoga, the mind and body, pain, attitude, patience, ego, sobriety, and the list could go on. I decided to mine that time for all the precious stones available. In each moment, there was a choice, particularly in my choices around how I treated my body and my perceptions about life and aging. On good days, my attitude was oriented toward recovery and well-being. To be rigorously honest, though, there were some days that were very painful and deeply depressing—just another reminder of my humanity and limitations. Today, when my back acts up (which it seems to do for whatever reason, like when I sneeze), I remember I get to choose how I relate to the experience one more time.

Anyone's here on their path is just another space in time during one's miraculous existence. The fact that we even exist in this vast universe is incredible, isn't it? In any given moment we can choose a path guided by the tenets of our spiritual life, provided we, as recovering people, want to dedicate ourselves to living a sober, conscious, and spiritual life. With this commitment, the task is then having a *progressively* clear definition of what recovery means, beyond quitting the drink, so we can consciously and actively move toward the recovery and life of well-being we envision. I like what one anonymous sober source said, "We must have a program for living that allows for limitless expansion."[2]

In moving toward the recovery we want, we make conscious choices. Then, the idea is to accept ourselves, others, and everything around us as is and see where our choices take us. We can always change course if we want and go as fast or as slow as the spirit guides. Looking forward at the horizon, having clarified a vision of who we want to be with ourselves, with others and with a Higher Power, we can move toward our ideal. We may not be able to see exactly where the path goes beyond the horizon, or what the end looks like, or if there really is an end. But that's okay.

What we do know about an end is that we will physically die someday.

We also know that if we betray our families or kill someone on the road drunk driving, this would certainly have an effect on others after we are gone.

But what about being in recovery and living a spiritual life of care and concern for ourselves and others? What about our legacy then? Will our children, grandchildren, friends, co-workers, or future generations glean any benefit from how we live our sober lives? I believe yes, but in precisely what ways we may never know. These are just a few of the unanswerable questions and great mysteries of life, don't you think?

To get sober is to get our life and all its mystery back. Using was a dead end for us addicts. We were the walking dead, and for some physically dead. Perhaps you know of someone who died or killed someone because of their addiction. What effect did it have on you? Or conversely, do you know anyone who died sober? If so, how did their life touch yours?

Many years ago, Jennifer, an acquaintance of mine in recovery, died of cancer. At Jennifer's memorial, a friend of hers shared what Jennifer had said to her on her death bed. The friend had asked Jennifer if there were any last words of wisdom she had to give. Jennifer said to her friend, "Never miss an opportunity to keep your mouth shut." I always chuckle when I remember this and have shared it countless times with many others who, like myself, have had the uncomely compulsion to correct the world into an image I want. It's like Jennifer bequeathed this delightful gift to all of us on that day, a gift that we can continue to give away. I doubt she knew this would be a gift that I would always treasure.

Sobriety requires living with a lot of unknowns. Not just the otherworldly or immeasurable unknowns but the unresolved matters we face in the here and now, every day. Having a feeling of satisfaction and well-being while not having answers about the status of a relationship, a job, a pet's illness, a business transaction, a child's destiny, a bad knee, or the exact time when the refrigerator repairman will show is a tall order for addicts. Throw in not having control over these people, places, things, and outcomes, and now we have a high potential for being swept into any one of several bad-feeling states. Most addicts want control. If we could just get a handle on these unknowns and outcomes, we would feel better, and so would everyone else!

Being in control is not necessarily a bad thing, but it sours when we try to control something outside of ourselves. There is a huge difference between having control and being controlling. Having control over what we can control—ourselves and our choices about everything—is a big part of what recovery is about.

Rather than attaching to something outside of ourselves for structure and comfort by attempting to control it, we can anchor to sound principles which teach us to focus on ourselves, do our part, let go, and then accept what is here, right now. This is being in recovery.

For many, the sober journey begins in a recovery program. What most addicts find is a much-needed support for living a sober, satisfied life. In the folds of this recovery care, we can calm down, wake up, and make sense of our lives. We awaken to our inner spirits, to others, and to a Higher Power, all available to guide us in recovery, healing, and transformation. Our hearts and minds can exist together in healthy, life-affirming ways.

The Recovery Cycle gives structure to the process of recovery. We can move from the grip of addiction to recovery and find a meaningful existence within our own unique, sober selves. We can discover people as sources of love in relationship. Even if a situation seems just awful, we can find satisfaction in doing the right thing if we stay sober and live by spiritual principles. I like to remember, "The spiritual life is not a theory. *We have to live it.*"[3]

With this information and all the other information and materials out there for recovery, an addict could spend the rest of his days growing in recovery. Each moment could be filled with something to work on. That said, it is not a good formula for a balanced life to be constantly working on oneself. Being in the wash cycle on agitate or spin indefinitely can be disastrous and is not what sober living is about. Keeping a sense of humor along with making time for play and recreational activities is part of a balanced life. Sure, we may grow up, but let's not forget to play. Have fun. Rest. Enjoy the fruits of your labor.

The Recovery Cycle provides a framework for sober living and loving. It is up to recovering individuals to delve honestly into their own hearts and minds to discover the spirit within as they find personal meaning in recovery and spiritual connection. With this new consciousness and a good dose of acceptance, these fortunate ones will be prepared to design their lives with purpose, reverence, and joy. These recovering people can be at home within and feel beautifully free.

Finally, this simple recovery plan is available to all who want it but can only be had by those who do it. For those who do it, life in recovery becomes a work of heart.

Notes

1   Viktor E. Frankl, *Man's Search for Meaning* (Boston: Beacon Press, 2006).
2   Alcoholics Anonymous., *Alcoholics Anonymous: Big Book Reference Edition for Addiction Treatment*, 4th ed. (New York: Alcoholics Anonymous, 2014), 275.
3   Ibid., 83.

Works Cited

Alcoholics Anonymous. *Alcoholics Anonymous: Big Book Reference Edition for Addiction Treatment*. 4th ed. New York: Alcoholics Anonymous, 2014.
Frankl, Viktor E. *Man's Search for Meaning*. Boston: Beacon Press, 2006.

Appendix

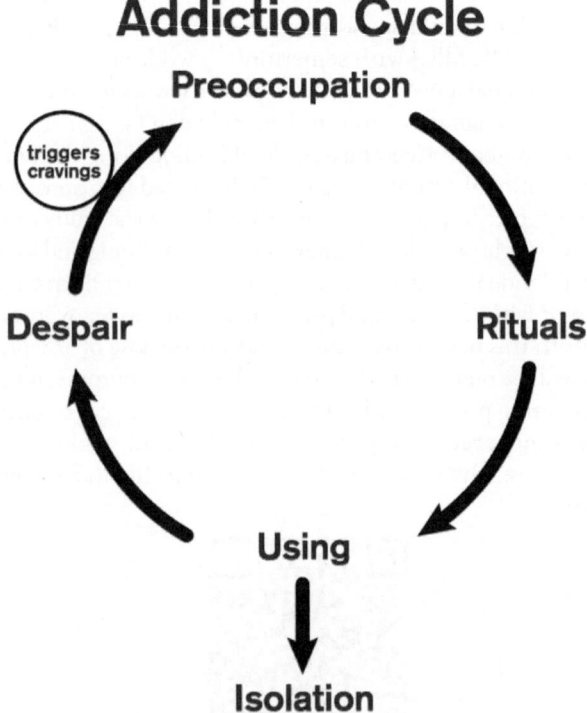

Figure A.1 The Addiction Cycle.

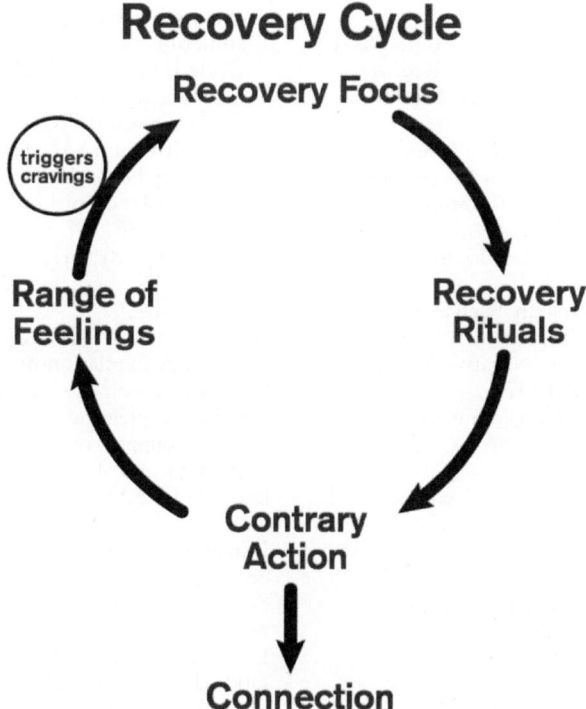

Figure A.2 The Recovery Cycle.

Index